Spirit
of the
Ancestors

Lessons from Africa

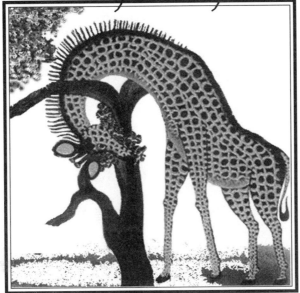

Susan Schuster Campbell

LOTUS
PRESS

P.O. Box 325, Twin Lakes, Wisconsin 53181

This book is a reference work, not intended to diagnose, prescribe or treat. The information contained herein is in no way to be considered as a substitute for consultation with a licensed health care professional. It is designed to provide information on traditional and historical folklore practices.

Cover and book design, page layout and composition by Susan Tinkle

First Edition 2002

Printed in the United States of America

Library of Congress Control Number : 2002108157
Campbell, Susan Schuster,
          Spirit of the Ancestors: Lessons from Africa
          ISBN   0 - 940985-37-3

Published by
Lotus Press, P.O. Box 325, Twin Lakes, Wisconsin 53181
email: lotuspress@lotuspress.com
website: www.lotuspress.com
1 (800) 824-6396

Ancestor: *noun* [C]
Ancestre from Latin *antecessor,*
literally "somebody who goes before"

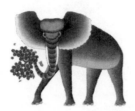

Human life is always guided,
it is balanced by your angel, your ancestor…
God works through your ancestors, my ancestors.

P.H. Mntshali,
Swazi Traditional Healer & Zulu Elder

May the nourishment of the Earth be yours,
May the clarity of light be yours,
May the fluency of the ocean be yours,
May the protection of the ancestors be yours
And so may a slow wind
warm these words of love around you,
forming an invisible cloak to mind your lives.

Irish blessing

Acknowledgements

I wish to thank my mentor and friend, P.H. Mntshali, who urged me to share the African experience through my Western eyes. I also thank those who generously shared their poignant anecdotes with me. Though I have remained true to your stories, some names have been changed to protect the privacy of clients where requested. Lastly, I am deeply grateful to and constantly inspired by my husband and son for their openness, support and laughter in the face of our adventurous lives. Their love has made this ancestral access even stronger.

Dedication

I dedicate this book to the ancestors who have worked so powerfully in my life, especially my paternal grandmother Catherine Farrell, my maternal grandfather Louis Kuptz, my father John "Jack" Schuster as well as my active in-laws, Joseph and Lillian "Lee" Campbell and the honorable Joseph Chapman Thompson.

May the veil between us always be thin.

Table of Contents

Preface

Thirty years later I can still see the picture clear as day. I had on my cook's uniform with a soiled apron. Dad wore a white dress shirt with the sleeves rolled up and a pair of dark suit trousers. I served him coffee and then relaxed against the ledge of the grill as we spoke. So began the story I told my mother.

My father was a traveling salesman who usually returned home on Friday evenings. This particular Friday I was at my part-time job at Woolworth's; when out of the blue, my father walked in and sat down at the lunch counter in front of me. He was home early and said he "just wanted to visit." He looked tired but seemed happy to be sitting there. He smiled often. I noticed the highlights in his gray hair and the pale sheen of his skin. I loved him so much in that moment and experienced such compassion for his effort to support our family of seven. Being with him felt different than other times though; it felt physical. It's hard to explain but if love could be a concrete sensation experienced in every inch of your body, well that is what I felt. I felt loved, protected, and unusually content.

"It was odd though," I told my mother, "during his visit I had no customers. Not a one, in fact we had no interruptions." This was extraordinary because a regular Friday crowd kept the place hopping. My mother was motionless as I told my story. Finally she said, "That is impossible. You started working at Woolworth's when you were fifteen years old. Remember?" Certainly, I remembered but what did she mean, "impossible?" "Susie," she continued, now calling me by my childhood name, "your father died when you were thirteen." Of course, I knew this in my bones. Yet, this contact two years after my father's death was no less real for me.

If my own family considered such natural contact with our deceased loved ones "impossible," how many others in our culture were rejecting benevolent attempts by ancestors to heal and guide us? Relationships continuing after death seemed so ordinary to me. If I could have such contact, so could they. For that matter, so could anyone.

Though ancestors had been part of my life since youth, it took an unusual relationship with African shamans many years later to harvest the assistance I was being offered. Like countless Americans, I had my life planned. A Vice-President of a prominent financial institution, with years of international consulting experience, I was well on my way to the top of the corporate ladder. Then I heard about the African healers and an unusual shift occurred.

In 1991, my family and I moved to southern Africa on an assignment. In the remoteness of the Kingdom of Swaziland, I began a journey away from my corporate world into one of spirituality and healing. Curious to learn more about the traditions of the Swazis, I accepted a rare invitation from the President of the Traditional Healers for Africa (THO) to visit him and a group of senior healers. The president, a personal healer to the King, oversaw an association of 20,000 members.

Exotic-looking people in feathers, beads and traditional clothing greeted me as I entered their offices. We chatted for hours, comparing our lifestyles and discussing family, spirituality and health. The healers shared their life view; that we are first and foremost, spiritual beings. God gives us a physical form in order that we may heal unfinished business and receive legacies gone unclaimed throughout our lineage. An unshakable belief in the spiritual intervention of the ancestors is the corner-stone of African tribal healing. As the healers said that day, "Nothing is impossible with the ancestors." Though our appearances indicated we lived in different worlds, our visit could not have been more comfortable or familiar.

Over the next seven years, I met with hundreds of master healers. My work with the healers gradually took priority. My family and I gained a new perspective through the process. We cherished life more and be-came more courageous. We made decisions that felt right at the time but didn't appear logical. Yet in the end, these choices resulted in the best move of our lives or the best job or the best place to live.

On my return home, I gave lectures on African healing but was soon responding to requests for practical workshops to apply the lessons I had learned. In a beautifully simple way, Africa offered another win-dow to our inner truths. Class participants who had never traveled to Africa, never met an African healer, or in some cases had no particular interest in African culture, began enthusiastically reporting success stories of their own using the simple practice of honoring their ancestors. Re-markably, they were finding answers to their modern problems using these traditions rooted in the past.

In the summer of 1999, my colleague, then 78 year-old Swazi Healer and Zulu Elder P.H. Mntshali, joined me in the USA for a lecture tour. We gave group presentations and consulted individually with hundreds of professionals in health, psychology, and spirituality as well as laypeople from all walks of life. We observed that Americans had lost access to their own ancestors. We listened to teachers, lawyers, hairdressers, entrepre-neurs, accountants, stay-at-home moms and dads, and others who sought this personalized spiritual assistance in their own modern lives. The idea of ancestors appealed to people of all lifestyles, cultures, and races. Con-tact with ancestors complemented a wide array of religious and spiritual practices.

At one of our last speaking engagements, P.H. Mntshali unexpect-edly announced, "Susan Schuster Campbell is exceptional in her abilities not only to understand and follow ancestral guidance, but also to share her own Western experience of this universal wisdom." I knew then, just as I knew years earlier, in that auspicious first meeting with the healers in remote Africa, that my next "assignment" was before me. It is my pleasure to share these stories and practices for our modern world in the hope that your own ancestors may find a place in your hearts.

CHAPTER ONE

Ancestral Communication: Our Spiritual Birthright

Opposites come to mind when I compare southern Africa and the United States. Our winter is their summer. We look to the future; Africans are oriented to the past. Many American families are small and self-sufficient, often separated from relatives by vast distances. Conversely, Africans have large extended families. Raising nephews and nieces while caring for one's own children and elderly relations is not uncommon. We guard our privacy and cherish peace and quiet. Africans often lead loud, boisterous communal lives. A friend of mine in Soweto, South Africa is fond of saying, "In Africa, if it's not worth shouting, it's likely not worth saying." However, our greatest difference may be found in how we view spirituality.

In the nine years my family and I lived in Swaziland, Botswana and South Africa, I was blessed to meet a cross-section of Africans from the illiterate and poor to highly placed executives with advanced degrees from Stanford and Oxford universities. This diverse population, representing a multitude of tribes, shared a common understanding of the importance of the spiritual in our daily lives. Access to a higher order of information and problem solving came to them through deceased loved ones, their *ancestors*. The ancestors acted as intermediaries to a higher consciousness, God. From time to time, they lost touch. Their spiritual communication was blocked and manifested itself as physical illness, emotional discomfort, or sheer bad luck. It was then time to call in the professional. They sought out their indigenous healer to make a strong spiritual contact on their behalf. The African healers lament a time when ordinary people were even better connected spiritually to their ancestors and naturally followed their inner guidance. Urbanization has propelled many of their clients into a faster, Western-style life. Their challenge, like ours, is to strengthen and maintain spiritual contact in daily life.

It is not only the mystical healer who has access to this powerful communication; rather it is the birthright of each and every human. This natural contact with the spiritual world is observed in the most ordinary life, in rural and urban Africa. I remember once taking an elevator in downtown Johannesburg. It was packed with corporate professionals on a busy weekday. As I pressed the floor number for my next meeting, I heard a woman from behind say, "No, no, you want floor fifteen." I turned but did not see anyone familiar. An African woman smiled at me and exited the next stop. She said, "fifteen" and stepped off. I had never seen this woman before.

There was nothing out of the ordinary about my appearance. I looked much like the others on the elevator. I had no papers out of my attaché case, no calling card with clues to my business in the building. Just for fun, I went to floor fifteen. Sure enough, the client I was visiting had moved offices since we last met two years earlier and was now located on floor fifteen. I mentioned the incident to my client, an American-educated African executive. She said, "Must have been the ancestors helping you through her."

While in Africa, I constantly observed a lack of self-consciousness where ancestral guidance was involved. In another incident, I attended a planning meeting at a national department in Pretoria. Discussing a variety of financing programs available for a new project, we went round the table soliciting final recommendations from senior officials. Administrative parameters of one program suggested a good fit; political constraints urged caution on another; one officer's Aunt had appeared in a dream the previous night and warned against a third program.

What? Someone's *dead aunt* had appeared in a dream with information? There was no laughing or teasing, which I might have expected in a Western setting such as this office. The information was noted and considered with the other contributions. In the end, we did not use the program the "auntie" cautioned against, as a better option was identified. The final decision was not based solely on the advice culled from the officer's dream but the spiritual information was simply accepted and added to the data.

Your lost loved ones are not dead, but gone before,
advanced a stage or two upon that road which you must travel
in the steps they trod.
                                                      – Aristophanes

---

Africans say that Westerners have many names for "ancestor;" forefather, ascendant, spirits, deceased, on the other side, angels, guides, supernatural beings, defender, benefactor, patron. Encarta World Dictionary 2001 says the word "Ancestor" originates from the Latin *antecedere*, which means simply "to go before." Those that have gone before are not limited in their communication to only African or indigenous peoples.

Thich Nhat Hanh, prominent Buddhist teacher and author, says that though we have blood ancestors we also have spiritual ancestors. For example, many of us born in the West are likely to have Jesus as our ancestor. Like the African mystics, the Buddhists consider Jesus as one of the many spiritual ancestors of Europeans. Though you may not consider yourself a Christian, your great-grandfather might have been a devout Christian. As an ancestor, he will transmit to you the seed, the love, and the insight of Jesus. You need only to tap into this energy to manifest this Christ love within yourself.

I myself was raised in the Roman Catholic Church. I attended parochial school in Wisconsin for the eight years of my elementary education. I learned about my guardian angel and put a name to the entity that seemed ever at my watch. Our loved ones who had moved on were also our intermediaries to God. My dreams were often vivid, with angels or loved ones showing me something I must do or understand. This seemed completely normal. So much so, that I do not recall talking about it with my parents or siblings. Ours was a busy household and an opportunity for such a discussion may not have presented itself. Still, talk of this nature seemed unnecessary, even trivial, in the natural order of my world.

I was graced with sensitive teachers, especially in my first few years. In the second grade I began to crave time alone in our church. Built like a small cathedral, Saint Mary's had stunning life-sized statues of Jesus, Mary and various saints throughout the building. This was a traditional time in the church. Mass was sung in Latin, ritual and ceremony abounded. I remember fondly the full acoustical sound of the organ, the high soprano voices of the choir, the richly embroidered robes of the priests, the clicking of rosary beads, and the swishing of the heavy black cloth of the habits of the Franciscan nuns.

Daily attendance at morning Mass was required at school but there was no opportunity to visit the church alone until Sister Ivo approached me. We children adored this exemplary and fun loving music teacher. One day she seemed to scoop me up as she took her typically long strides down the hallway. Grabbing my hand she walked me to her classroom and together we quickly set up the chairs. In the moment before the other children entered, Sister Ivo said, "Did you know that the eighth grade girls clean the church when it is empty? You may help them today." The room quickly filled with my classmates and I could barely contain my excitement.

During our afternoon recess, I ran to meet the older girls at the church. I was to dust my favorite statues. Much to my surprise, the girls soon left to tidy the priests' changing rooms. I could not believe my luck; I was completely alone. I soaked in the residual smell of the heavy frankincense and myrrh, the brightness of the vigil candles at the side shrines, and the exquisite and ancient looking murals of ascending bodies on the ceiling above the main altar. I laid back in a pew, held my arms straight out from my body and prayed silently, "thank you, God."

In the next instant, I heard a soft voice and sat up sharply. Lying around in the church was a serious offense and would surely jeopardize any future visits with the cleaning crew. I heard the soft voice again, almost a whisper, from behind, this time saying only "come." I looked around and noticed the statue of Mother Mary with her arms outstretched. I rushed over and lay back against the statue, extending my arms so they fit on top of her shoulders. The time had an exceptional quality. I did not feel rushed. I was unconcerned about the older girls returning and finding me in this position. In fact, it seemed I could stay there safely forever. In that seminal moment I felt spirituality as a natural and necessary life force, quite separate from religion or dogma.

I don't remember walking away from the statue but I next heard one of the older girls ask me, "Are you finished now?" I felt my feather duster drop to the floor. The girls helped me gather up my duster and supplies. I thought it odd that they didn't speak sharply as was typical when dealing with us younger ones. During my remaining years at St. Mary's, Sister Ivo always had a private wink for me when we passed in the hall and allowed me access to the church from time to time.

Adolescence challenged my spiritual experiences as schoolmates mocked contact with angels and ancestors. Following my father's death, I entered public high school and found further ways to suppress my embarrassing spiritual connection. Leaving home for university proved a godsend, introducing me to people of different faiths, race, and culture. Vestiges of the 1960's left minds opened to Eastern mysticism, philosophy, meditation, yoga, and natural healing. Contact with spirits beyond our physical space was no longer absurd and even scientists were exploring guidance of a higher nature.

I wondered if having successfully blocked out much of this contact for years, I'd ever experience it again. You can imagine my surprise when at nineteen years old, my father appeared in a dream and instructed me to find books by an Elisabeth Kubler-Ross. I had never heard of this author, yet my father showed me how her unusual name was spelled. The next morning I woke with a vivid memory of the dream. I attended classes but the name Kubler-Ross kept running through my mind. I stopped at the library on the way home to my dormitory. I started reading *On Death and Dying* that night. The book was insightful and helped me not only put to rest my father's passing, but also to restore my conscious contact with him and others.

> "Tradition is a guide and not a jailer."
>
> – W. Somerset Maugham

In the early 1900's, my family of German and Irish ancestry felt pressure to discard our own legacies to better fit into mainstream America. Like so many others of their time, ancestral languages, traditions, and rituals were suppressed and eventually forgotten. Nonetheless, with little knowledge and often no photographs, I was surprised at the ease with which ancestors made contact with me.

For example, both my grandmothers whom I had never known appeared in dreams with information that was specifically useful at the time. My father's mother Catherine has been particularly active in my dreams and thoughts whenever a concern about my son arises. Like me, she had one child, a son. She died when my father was a toddler. I am the first person in my father's family to have had only one child. I often feel Catherine Farrell's legacy and support as I raise my son. Often I put questions to her that fall outside my extended family's experience. Consistently I receive a thoughtful response that moves me from worry or confusion to peace.

> "Death ends a life, not a relationship."
>
> – Tuesdays with Morrie

During our 1999 tour, my Zulu colleague and I discussed and described communication with ancestors as understood in the African context and mirrored in my own personal experiences. Our audiences cited current references within popular culture. They named films such as the "Field of Dreams" where the character played by actor Kevin Costner is told by "ancestors" to build a baseball field on his good agricultural land; the Bruce Willis film "The Sixth Sense" where a young boy has the ability not only to communicate with the dead but to help resolve unfinished business. The films "Hearts & Souls," "Déjà vu," and others were noted.

Current books topping the bestseller lists included several that explored ways to reach and receive help from the other side. A line from the popular book, *Tuesdays with Morrie* by Mitch Albom, was much quoted, "Death ends a life, not a relationship." In a 1994 USA Today-CNN-Gallop poll, nearly 70 million Americans said they think it is possible to communicate with the dead. Spiritual encounters like mine, which occur when we are contacted directly and spontaneously by a loved one who has passed on, without the use of psychics or mediums, had even been labeled After-Death Communication or ADC by researchers in the USA and Canada.

Business Week magazine gave top coverage to an exploding spirituality in America, which included indigenous ancestral practices, eastern meditation and traditional religious observations. "Today, a spiritual revival is sweeping across Corporate America as executives of all stripes are mixing mysticism into their management. When companies engage in programs that use spiritual techniques for their employees, productivity improves and turnover is greatly reduced."[1]

Curiosity about ancestors was an important factor in a new trend amongst our children. "Education abroad is rapidly expanding, bolstered by an increasing number going to explore their ethnic roots. More American college students went overseas in 1999 to study than ever before, according to a survey released Monday by the Institute of International Education."[2]

Our ancestors would find this renewed attention to lineage, spirituality and mysticism truly an appropriate time to strengthen our ancestral contact and claim their assistance. Our communication with them is no "far-out" mystical experience but rather our natural birthright. No great mystery to be solved before reaching them, no complicated procedures to gain access, but rather a simple return, a "tuning-in" to the ancestors' subtle wavelengths.

---

[1] "The Growing Presence of Spirituality in Corporate America," *Business Week* Magazine, November 1999

[2] "Tide of U.S. Collegians Studying Abroad Swells: a search for ethnic roots," *Los Angeles Times*, November 15, 2000

CHAPTER TWO

Prepare for Contact: Turn Your Radio On

In rural Africa, telephones are so scarce that information must be relayed by radio. The local stations often broadcast personal and public messages in the evening. A person may have a radio but if it is not turned on, communication falls on deaf ears. Likewise, our ancestral spirits may be passing information to us but if we are not aware, if we do not have our own "radios" on, we'll miss the contact.

A wonderful way to turn on our radios, to initiate or renew ancestor contact, is through a celebration. In African and other indigenous traditions, an annual commemoration is typical. Annual honoring of the dead is found in religious customs as well, such as All Souls' Day in Roman Catholic churches in America or the Day of the Dead in Mexico. People of the Jewish faith honor their ancestors on the anniversary of the ancestor's death and during Yom Kippur.

My Asian friends have small altars in their homes adorned with flowers and photographs of their ancestors. These provide a special place to make daily contact with their ancestors. By honoring loved ones who have passed, we initiate or refresh our spiritual contact with them. Through them, we also strengthen our contact with the greater divine conscious-ness, God, the Creator, Buddha or Allah for whom the ancestors act as intermediaries. Once opened or renewed, this contact is a powerful source of ongoing support and insight.

If you do not have a tradition of your own, try my favorite ancestor party based on an old African custom. After all, many scientists believe that man first appeared on earth in Africa. Therefore, everyone has Afri-can ancestors; all the more reason to give it a try.

Ancestor Party

The ancestor party should suit your circumstances and inclinations. It may be elaborate and involve many invited guests or be a simple meal taken alone. You may prefer a breakfast or brunch rather than an evening meal. The meal may be an informal picnic at a grassy park, a gathering in your kitchen or a formal dinner party. Your sincere *intent* to honor your ances-tors is more important than the physical aspects of the event. Once given, the ancestor honoring can become a wonderful annual event. My family gives such a party at the beginning of every year. It fits nicely with other celebrations and the general holiday spirit found that time of year in the Western world. Choose dates and times that have personal signifi-cance for you.

In addition to this annual event, I am often moved to give special attention to individual ancestors throughout the year. For instance, for years I gave a special recognition meal for my father. I usually remem-bered to do this in January, his birthday month. One year I was traveling and forgot. It didn't occur to me again until April. I looked at my calendar and the 22nd was an open day for me. I prepared a simple meal and enjoyed it with my family while sharing stories about him. The following year I also "forgot" in January and found myself thinking of my father more strongly in April. In an unrelated conversation with my mother, as we compared calendars to arrange a visit, she reminded me that my father had died on April 22, 1965. Though I had been celebrating on or near his birthday, now the remembrance event shifted to and remains in April, the month of his passing. Likewise you too will be drawn to dates and times that have personal meaning or simply appeal. The significance of the timing may only be revealed later. Either way, follow your feeling and enjoy the event, small or large.

Ring the bells that still can ring
Forget your perfect offering.
There is a crack in everything
That's how the light gets in.

-Leonard Cohen

Do not worry about your celebration being a "perfect offering." Your effort will be appreciated because it is yours, just right in its entirety. The spirit world is light and enjoys laughter and fun. As you prepare for your ancestor party, think of your lineage. What music evokes their ethnicity? What foods represent their heritage? What fragrances bring them to mind? What tablecloths and dishware would you use if your ancestors were physically able to visit this day? It is not important whether you actually knew them in life. If you were adopted, call forward both your birth lineage (which may or may not be known to you) and the lineage of your adopted family. These families have deep connections spiritually. Invite the ancestors to join together in this feast commemorating their roles in your lives.

As you plan, images, foods, music, and scents will be suggested to you. One of my clients recently had her first ancestor party. The various details came together beautifully though she was stumped on what to wear. Finally, the morning of her dinner she was drawn to a bright yellow dress. Although a more formal outfit seemed appropriate she could not deny her attraction to this simple dress. She wore the dress and was at ease throughout the party. Several weeks later she wore the same dress to a family reunion. At the gathering, an elder aunt approached her, very touched by both the style and color of the dress. Unbeknownst to my client, she is the descendent of a great aunt who wore the same style dress. Yellow was her favorite color. There were other similarities as well. It seems, this ancestor "communicated" to my client, very well.

Dressing the Ancestors

In the African tradition, a piece of white fabric of a natural fiber symbolizes the "dress" of the ancestors. The cloth is dedicated to the ancestors through a thoughtful prayer or meditation, a heartfelt wish, your intent. Place the cloth in the middle of the table as a runner, tablecloth or decoration. I use a thirty-year-old white cotton cloth embroidered on the edges by my mother-in-law. Lee and I were very close and after her death, the cloth was left uncompleted. Later, my father-in-law remarried and his new wife, as a surprise to us, finished the embroidery and presented it as a gift to my family. Marlene's action was an exquisite symbol of stitching our families together. The cloth always had a sacred feel. With this added significance, it was perfect for ancestor parties.

Ancestor parties are an ordinary part of African life, but they may be the exception in our culture. Should this be the case with you, remember that intent is key. The first time I invited outside guests to an ancestor party, I worried that I might offend or inhibit with my strange custom. An ancestor party must be done graciously and with love. It is critical that those attending feel welcome and comfortable. It is a day we embrace humankind and demonstrate kindness. With this in mind, I decided to create the experience in an unobtrusive manner. I invited guests to dinner but did not specifically call it an ancestor party.

I cooked the foods that honored our lineage and evoked special memories, placed ancestral and family photographs subtly throughout the house, played Irish and German music for my family's side as well as Scottish and Scandinavian music to honor my husband's lineage. I lit fragrant candles, and prepared, as usual. It was a cozy and comfortable event. Guests asked questions about artifacts, photographs, music and food that inevitably prompted stories about our ancestors. Through the stories, we discovered new links with our guests. The conversation was lively. There was an unusual appetite for family stories. So you see, if your intent is sincere and heartfelt, your party will be perfect, however it unfolds.

Ancestors and unseen guiding spirits around us today, please bless us as you join together to reach us in your healing effort. May we have the courage to listen with our hearts, and to suspend our demanding logic. Please accept our pure intent and make us better instruments in this, our modern world.

-Schuster Campbell Family "Ancestor Party Prayer"

Traditionally, the male lineage is asked to lead and extend a welcome to relations on the other side of the family. In our annual family ancestor party, we acknowledge my father-in-law who passed away recently, and his lineage. We ask that they extend a welcome to my mother-in-law's family and then to my entire lineage. We acknowledge that our families were brought together to further facilitate growth and healing. It is a time to respect their attempts to resolve any weaknesses and special challenges they may have faced while in physical form. Their efforts, however grand or minor, have affected our own legacy.

If you are unmarried, call forward your father and his side of the family in a similar fashion. Request that his line greet and include your mother's side. There may have been differences, even hate between parties while they lived. This disparity is often the stuff of great, even humorous stories when seen through the light of love and compassion. Abandon your belief system regarding these people before death.

A friend of mine reported vivid dreams the night of her first ancestor celebration. Though she was leery and thought my idea "a little kooky" she was intrigued enough to try her own variety of commemoration. She rang me the next day, agitated that "the wrong" ancestor had visited her. She described a drunken uncle, who had eventually died succumbing to his alcoholism. This "contact" was perceived as a slap in the face, especially given her own challenge with substance abuse.

This did not surprise me. What better ancestor to make contact than one with unfinished business surrounding addiction? Over time, this ancestor appeared in several dreams and helped my friend at decisive moments in her own successful recovery. The ancestors' struggles and talents can be of equally valuable help. During your celebration, suspend your preconceived notions, show respect, reminisce in good humor and enjoy the occasion.

Reporting to the Ancestors

A report of the past year is always given before the meal is eaten. Briefly detail the challenges and blessings of the past year and express gratitude for the ancestors' intercession on one's behalf. Lastly, we ask for help in those areas we need it most. Again, tailor your reporting to fit your needs, heritage and situation. Some prefer a spokesperson give the greeting and report in their names. Others, like my family, prefer to invite each present to say a few words, adding to the total report. In the above example with our outside guests, I asked my husband to say grace. In the prayer, Ron gave a brief overview of our year, gave thanks and asked for divine assistance. The theme of family and thanksgiving had emerged so naturally in the pre-dinner conversation that several guests added touching words of their own.

Feeding the Ancestors

Many cultures have a tradition of remembering the deceased with a physical gesture, such as offering food or drink. At the strike of New Year's for example, my family drops a bit of drink on the front doorstep to toast with our Irish and Scottish ancestors. Such ritual is also part of the ancestor party. Depending on your preferences, you might put a symbolic place setting for the ancestors at the table or simply raise a glass to offer a toast on their behalf. I place small tastes of each food on the plate. Upon completion of the meal, I put the plate in my garden for the birds and cats. In keeping with the day's atmosphere of hospitality, no food should be left uneaten. Give parting guests leftovers to take home. This is a gesture our own ancestors used in their lifetimes and is still cherished today.

It is believed that the ancestors may send unexpected guests to your door when an ancestor party is underway. On this day, none should be turned away. Unanticipated family, neighbors, or guests should be greeted warmly and invited into the gathering. The ambiance of the event is lovely and has its own special way of calling forward the best behavior and results, even after the event.

In 1980, my husband and I were on our first assignment in Africa. Living in the small, isolated mining town of Selebi-Phikwe, Botswana, we decided to have an intimate ancestor party and invite a group of colleagues and neighbors to join us immediately afterwards. The legendary President Seretse Khama led the country. Married to a white English woman, this first family was a shining example of equality amongst races during some of the darkest years of apartheid in neighboring South Africa. Even so, emotion ran high across racial lines.

Our neighbors, an older Afrikaner couple, returned our daily greetings and smiles with silence and frowns. Our professional lives naturally included many Africans as well as East Indians, Asians and others working and living in this developing community. Our conservative neighbors were avid supporters of the divided system of apartheid. They let us know we were headed for trouble associating with such a mixed crowd. On the day of our party, we quietly enjoyed our own small ancestor meal then awaited our invited guests. Before long we had sixty people overflowing our small Town Council house spilling into the backyard in full view of our stony neighbors. They had not accepted our invitation. The music was wonderful and the mood a special treat prompting new friendships across color and economic lines.

The next morning I was surprised at my door by my neighbor holding the cutest little puppy. He handed me the puppy as a "gift of friendship." He invited my husband and me to have a meal with him and his wife. He noticed "what good fun" we seemed to be having at the previous day's party. He hoped he and his wife would have an opportunity to attend the next time. Even though we had hosted previous social functions at our residence, they detected some special feeling about the gathering, which prompted them to come closer. While we remained distanced philosophically, we did have dinner with our neighbors and opened an ongoing dialogue of our respective experiences and beliefs.

Dreaming with the Ancestors

The night of the ancestor party is an excellent time to make dream contact with your special guardians and helpers. Take the special white cloth you used from the table and put it under your pillow or if large enough, you can even sleep directly upon it. It is the *symbolic gesture* of the cloth, which is important, and your *intent* to be a clear communication instrument for dream contact. Before sleep, report again to your ancestors. Give thanks for their support. Petition their assistance by asking that the ancestor most appropriate to help you in this current phase of your life make contact. Upon waking, take just a moment to jot first impressions, fragments of the dream, first thoughts that come to mind. This may be important and helpful information. Now that the contact, no matter how subtle, has been established, it is important to maintain. Keep those radios on. Keep your reception strong.

CHAPTER THREE

Getting Better Reception:
Slow Down, Prioritize, Simplify

Africans say we are energetic in our spiritual laziness. We fill our lives with compulsive activity and soon our lives are "living" us. Unimportant tasks or so-called responsibilities consume our daily routines and we disconnect from our spiritual center. We forget that this life is lived in an instant. We must be clear on our priorities or risk this precious "instant" slipping through our fingers. The healers suggest a simple remedy for our fast-paced modern lives. When life is moving too fast; when there are too many demands on our lives; when we are tipping toward chaos; there is but one remedy, one response. We must slow down to regain our focus, to reactivate our contact with ancestral guidance.

You must learn to be still in the midst of activity,
and to be vibrantly alive in repose.

– Indira Ghandi

Before we can truly observe the nuances and notice the subtleties of spiritual and ancestral communication, we must find or consciously create unhurried moments in our busy schedules to center ourselves. A colleague once asked, "If you could describe life in the U.S.A. in one word, what would it be?" Without hesitation, I answered, "distracting." I could also have said that at times it can be excessive or fast but "distracting" sums it up. Returning to the U.S.A., I realized how different my life had been in the developing world. Whether living in Africa, the South Pacific or Central Europe, I needed simply to open my door and walk outside to be reminded that I was not in my own culture. I learned not to make assumptions and developed an art of asking questions and seeking clarification in all my interactions, personal and professional. The environment demanded I pay attention to information coming through all my senses. It prevented me from judging too quickly and caused me to be in the present, as much as possible.

These cultures each have what I have come to think of as built-in "slowing down" mechanisms. Greeting someone on the street, for instance, is a long process, asking after the person's family, health, and spiritual well being. Entering an office for a business meeting, one starts with this same greeting followed by drinking tea together. In a grocery store or at the market, the vendor or cashier is greeted or "recognized" before the purchase transaction begins. In the Zulu language, this greeting translates literally to "I see you." I acknowledge and honor you.

There are similar customs for leave taking as well. In Poland, for example, one announces as much as one hour prior to departure that you must leave. This signals to the group or individual with whom you are visiting that it is time to complete the visit and discuss or say anything of importance.

Taking time to be quiet is the best gift you can give yourself.

– Oprah

In our Western culture, slowing down takes more of an effort. Stepping off that constant treadmill of activity usually requires a conscious act such as a meditation practice. I have tried a variety of meditation techniques in the past, but have been put off by practices that seemed complicated, grueling, or not in sync with my spiritual beliefs. I felt a revelation when I read author Robert Thurman, "The first type of meditation you can begin with is the calming meditation, called one-pointedness. You practice in short sessions, five or ten minutes at a time, starting with observing your breaths, counting them, relaxing and calming, letting your thoughts go their own way without dragging you with them. Always stop the sessions while you are enjoying them. Never prolong them until you are tired. The idea is to condition yourself to enjoy them and to want to go back to them." Meditation need not necessarily be an arduous exercise.

I also enjoy walking meditation, which is being quietly aware of each step I take, conscious of the plants I pass, the people and animals I encounter, mindful of the fragrances and colors presented along the way. Another effortless but effective practice is to bring to mind an image that conveys tranquility. At times I visualize the face of a loved one, or a favorite setting in nature, or a sacred icon. It never fails to help calm my nerves when distressed. A meditation I like to use with audiences to tenderly jog their observation powers is the Raisin Meditation.

Find a quiet place to sit uninterrupted for several minutes. Take one small raisin in your hand. Notice its dry, hard shape. Now place it in your mouth and close your eyes. Do not bite or chew the raisin. Notice what is happening inside your mouth. You are salivating and the hard, flat piece of fruit is starting to feel different on your tongue. The raisin is becoming more plump and soft. Now bite into the raisin. Observe the explosion of taste. Such a simple exercise is a quick reminder of the importance of our observation proficiency. When we observe and judge too quickly, we often miss the important spiritual message or clue. If we dismiss an ancestral instruction at first glance, we may miss a golden opportunity. If I learned one thing from my African mystic friends, it is that everything matters. Each feeling, dream, thought, observation, in short, anything we notice has meaning and is designed to draw us closer to our genuine calling, keep us on our path to our legacies.

These simple techniques help me return to that uncomplicated African time when every encounter with the environment and culture served as a gentle reminder to pay attention, to return to a deeper spiritual nature. Slowing down does not necessarily have to come through a conscious meditation. It can be found in the simple tasks we perform repeatedly. For example, my husband asked me to iron his shirts. He wasn't happy with our laundry service. I volunteered to help out until we could find a dry cleaner to our liking. My mother happened to call the next day and I mentioned the dreaded ironing ahead. My mother was perplexed. "I love ironing. Are you sure you don't like it?" I was surprised to hear this from an active senior citizen who still held down a job and was too busy with friends and family to do much ironing herself.

My mother was forty-three years old when my father's death left her alone with five children. She did not have a job and was unaccustomed to handling the family financial resources. My siblings and I worked after school babysitting, mowing lawns, and flipping burgers. It was a struggle to make ends meet and I remember how tired my mother was, coming home from her full-time job. Yet, she would wait for us children to go to bed, and then set up her ironing board.

It was hardest, she said, to iron that first shirt but she would soon find herself noticing pleasure like the warmth of the steam coming from the iron on a cold Wisconsin winter night. Then, she would notice whose shirt it was she was ironing, and remember how proud he was to choose that shirt himself, how fond he was of it. She would begin to give extra care to the collar and the button down front, making it all crisp and fresh. Finally she would hang the shirt up, admire the shirt and imagine the child in it, and stand back and feel so full of love and so very blessed. By the end of the evening and the bottom of her laundry basket, she said she didn't know why, but she felt less tired and closer to God.

The meaning of things lies not in the things themselves,
but in our attitude towards them.

– Antoine de Saint Exupery

Africans perceive Westerners as "too" willing to exchange opportunity, life experience and ancestral quests for comfort and consumerism.

The Africans, being sophisticated in a highly developed age-old barter system, believe this is a poor trade indeed. There is no mistaking that we value our possessions. Inherently, there is nothing wrong with material things. The heartbreak comes only when priorities are askew and the quality of our relationships and lives are compromised to acquire these objects. Janet Luhrs, a lawyer and publisher of *Simple Living Journal* in Seattle says, "Time, freedom and serenity - there is no way you can have those if you're on a treadmill of work and spend. Nobody's advocating going broke. The object is to make money and possessions work for you instead of against you."

Having moved across oceans and set up house in all variety of environments, I know full well how little we actually "need" to have a happy, well functioning home, even in America. Moving has provided many wonderful occasions to cull my worldly goods. I relate easily to people who live in small spaces such as boats, trailers, condos, trucks, or apartments because every new item brought home is better received if it has a purpose and fits an available space. Shopping with these discerning people is such a pleasure. They have to really love the item to bring it home. For the nomads amongst us, we must not only love the item but it must be easy to transport as well.

My first overseas assignment was as a Peace Corps Volunteer in the South Pacific in the mid-1970's. I spent one of my two years on an island that had no vehicles, roads, running water, electricity, radio communication, or medical clinic. My home was a hut built of bush materials set upon stilts. When I asked for a window in my one-room house, the villagers happily slashed several with their machetes. Though my house was situated on a nearly inaccessible bay, occasionally an experienced yacht made its way through. I fondly remember conversations with visiting Australian and American adventurer families, extolling our good fortune to be without so many "conveniences." Living this way helped me to re-evaluate. I can live without many electronic devises for instance, but a washing machine became precious after years of doing laundry by hand.

My family and I have yielded, with delight, to those consumer urges each time we are living back home and have a little larger space but we do know that given an open heart and the right ancestral urge, leaving it all behind is not nearly as difficult as one might imagine.

My mother-in-law was diagnosed with lymphoma cancer while my husband and I were overseas in the mid-1980's. We made a difficult decision to quit our jobs and return to Seattle to be closer to Lee. We had faced ambiguity before and knew that logistics, including new sources of income, would unfold. We had one full, rich year with Lee in which we presented her with a new grandson. Ron and I settled into exciting jobs and our son grew into a happy preschooler.

One evening, long after Lee had died and her surviving loved ones were well into their new lives, we relaxed around our dinner table. We were living the American dream, complete with first-rate jobs and the requisite dream house, with decks and views of the ocean and mountains at every turn. Ron began musing about taking our son, then 4 years old, to Africa. Joseph would love the African culture and outdoor lifestyle. He would see how "the other half lives." Rather than our teaching compassion in theory, Joseph would be immersed in situations where his love for humanity would naturally blossom.

That spontaneous conversation shifted my perception of my surroundings. I knew in that instant that I would gladly trade our comfort and security for a family adventure in Africa. A family exploration "felt" considerably more important than any career advancement or additional assets or bigger and better vacations. Within a year, we had sold our house and were on a plane to our new "home" in Swaziland with one very excited little boy.

Simplicity is the ultimate sophistication

– Leonardo Da Vinci

I urge you to prioritize what is important in your world. Be ruthlessly honest with yourself, it's your life at stake. Recognize what and who is truly vital to you. Keep possessions in their proper perspective. With less physical clutter and fewer demands from unnecessary or negative people in your circle, you will be surprised how clearly those ancestral promptings begin reaching you. Find your own practice for slowing down the mind. Look hard at the priorities in your life. Simplify your environment; lose the clutter both physical and psychological. Your "reception" to the ancestors will improve greatly. You will be better prepared to act when the contact comes.

CHAPTER FOUR

Making Contact

Ancestral contact often starts with one main ancestor, your own "guardian spirit," who will endeavor to contact you through all your senses, including your intuition. A fragrance we smell reminds us of someone we would like to visit. We stop over only to find he has an unexpected houseguest who helps us. A dream suggests action; a song's lyrics give us a helpful lesson; or we are drawn to accept or resist certain invitations. We crave foods that turn out to have been favorites of the particular ancestor trying to make contact. We're attracted to colors or garments that prove reminiscent of them. Responding to these desires and impulses bring the ancestors closer, allowing them to communicate. Do not try to apply logic to these urges, simply be willing to act on them. You will be surprised where these seemingly small steps will take you.

Human life is always guided, it is balanced by your angel, your ancestor. People now are so learned, so willful. They forget that they go with a guide who they must obey. I see people who have lost touch. They say they live by God but their actions show otherwise. God is the big boss but He works with ancestors, your ancestors, my ancestors.

–P.H. Mntshali, from *Called to Heal*

In my youth ancestral contact first came as an expression, a strong communication of love such as in the incident of my father visiting me at the Woolworth's lunch counter after his death. At nineteen years old, my father still remained my "main ancestor" and he began to offer specific instruction such as when he referred me to Dr. Kubler-Ross' book. Later his mother, my grandmother Catherine, appeared in my dreams. I was forty years old the first time it happened. I had thought of Catherine just before sleep. I had no question to ask her, so merely said a short thank you for her influence in my life. That evening I had a dream of my grandmother showing me a jacket I must give a friend. I was surprised to see Catherine and taken aback when she told me to give away my favorite jacket.

In the dream I was seeing Catherine as if in peripheral vision. I was not paying complete attention to her words as I tried to quickly move my head to see her more clearly. My grandmother admonished me and said her *message* was vital, not her image. As early as her first dream contact, she cautioned me to focus on the message, not the phenomena of seeing her in my sleep. Later she was to give me instruction with only words and no visuals, then only subtle feelings and no words.

The day after this dream I did give my friend the jacket. She was ecstatic. Unbeknownst to me, she had just received an invitation to speak at an international conference. She had no time to shop and was desperate to find such a jacket that traveled well. It was payment enough to see her so happy. Additionally, she met contacts at the conference that later proved very useful in my own work. In retrospect we both admitted we could not have scripted the turn of events any better ourselves.

Synchronicity increases when we follow or even simply pay attention to any "message" received. Notice recurring thoughts you are having. Pay attention to overheard conversations that seem especially meant for you. Be aware of people, places, music, pictures, fragrances, and food you are being drawn to. Observe and watch the message unfold. It is not always clear why the ancestors ask us to do certain things and this can be maddening, given our Western sensibilities. However, accompanying the communication is often a feeling of volition. An action is called for and we are drawn to it in subtle ways.

For example, I had been toying with the idea of expanding my speaking engagements from health care professionals to a broader audience. I knew an ongoing spiritual, ancestral connection was possible in any walk of life. We are born with a divine connection and need not defer to psychics, mystics or mediums. In addition to my own experience, I had witnessed this connection with very ordinary people across Africa but I wanted stories from my own culture. I wanted a story of a typical middle-class modern American responding to a call. Prior to sleep one evening I asked for corroboration, perhaps just one story which might sanction my desire to reach out to a lay audience. The answer came quickly and in a surprising manner.

The next morning I woke with the thought, "Go to Costco." Costco is my neighborhood warehouse-shopping club. Truly an American phenomenon, it stocks bulk quantities of quality merchandise at wholesale prices. I loved the whole Costco shopping experience. The aisles were wide and merchandise well organized. Fellow shoppers came prepared with long lists and focused on the job at hand. The stockroom setting, stripped of all but the essentials, made it easy to concentrate. Spending much of my adult life in the developing world, access to goods and services such as Costco offered, still seemed exceptional. I completely appreciated the availability and wide selection of goods. However, shopping for my family required only one trip a month, which I had just made. I had no list, nothing to buy. Still, the idea of going to Costco stayed with me. I finally surrendered and cancelled my plans for the morning.

Arriving at Costco, I took a shopping cart and strolled around the building. I paid attention to what I noticed, new books, boys' clothing, and produce, nothing unusual. Time passed and I soon felt the urge to leave. Though I had nothing to show for my excursion, I felt satisfied. My divine "task" seemed finished. Just then I became aware of a woman in her mid-thirties with a small blonde-headed cherub in her cart. As I glanced at the boy, his mother said, "I love your hair cut." I noticed her hair as well. Like mine, it was very short. We laughed about hair, its short length being in direct proportion to the increased demands on our lives. She then told me a story.

A corporate executive, she returned to her firm following maternity leave after her son's birth. Her work in finance was exhilarating. She was challenged and enlivened by it. Nonetheless, each day she found her thoughts drifting back to her son and her home. This took her by surprise. She diagnosed it as a mild but lingering symptom of post-partum depression. As the days turned into months, she found her career satisfaction waning. In spite of a promotion, new clients and exciting portfolio prospects, the thrill seemed to be gone.

Working part-time might be an option. She explored this scenario with her husband who also felt she needed a change. The possibility of forfeiting half her income caused them to reconsider their expenses. They could manage nicely, albeit without some of the extras to which they had become accustomed. They agreed. She would explore part-time work.

To her own surprise, she walked into her boss' office and said, "I want to resign." Odd as the words sounded, she said, "They felt true, as if my soul were speaking to me. I felt it was a call. It felt, and still feels, so right." Since that day two years ago, she has been a full-time, stay at home mom. She told me of the many, many adjustments she and her husband had made to facilitate this change. From a major relocation to a more modest neighborhood to finding inexpensive haircuts, she remained invigorated by the transformation of their lifestyle.

She and her son were very relaxed with each other. It was a delight to hear her story and see them together. In parting she said, "I'm not in the practice of opening up to strangers and certainly not about this 'call' of mine, but when I saw you, I kept having the thought to tell you this story. I hope you don't mind." I thanked her profusely and told her how I happened to be there. Her story was my affirmation, the sanction to expand beyond healing professionals to embrace people of all walks of life.

My words are so easy to understand,
So easy to follow,
And yet nobody in the world
Understands or follows them.

Words come from an ancestry,
Deeds from mastery:
When these are unknown, so am I.

- Tao Te Ching

Early in one's experience with ancestors, it is easy to magnify and complicate what may be just simple direction. Frequently we are offered a slight adjustment, a little nudge, rather than a thunderbolt or complete life change as the following story illustrates. Culled from my husband's days as a Divinity student in college, the following story rings true for communication from the ancestors as well.

A farmer was distressed to see his wheat crop failing. He spent sleepless nights worrying that he would not be able to provide for his family. In desperation he prayed to God and asked for a sign, some indication of what he must do to survive. The next day the farmer felt calmer and worked peacefully in his fields. Suddenly clouds formed overhead. In giant letters, the clouds spelled out "GPC." The farmer fell to the ground and thanked God for such a clear sign. There could be no doubt, God wanted him to forsake this farming business and of course, *Go Preach Christ.* The request felt odd to him, his heart was not in such work but then again, who was he to second-guess God?

Though the farmer had neither training nor inclination toward preaching, he took on his newfound "calling" with forced enthusiasm. He began preaching to any group of people who were willing to listen and soon found himself a small following. As time marched on, the farmer-preacher struggled to understand and address the needs of his few faithful. His income in this new venture was inadequate and he missed his intimacy with the earth. In a moment of depression he asked God, "Why did you ask me to preach when in my heart, I am a humble farmer?" Suddenly a clear voice whispered, "I said GPC, Go Plant Corn."

Such is the humor of our attempts to make spiritual direction grandiose and dramatic. True, there are moments when we are advised to stretch outside our routine lives but more often than not; we are asked to make many minor adjustments as we take baby steps toward mysticism.

Khumbulile Mdluli, a Swazi healer, explains: "when a thought comes to my mind, and keeps coming back, I know it is guidance from my ancestors. My ancestors told me where to build my clinic and how it should look. I follow my ancestors correctly and exactly. With modernization and change in lifestyle, people begin to see this contact with their ancestors as something primitive. They ignore the attempts of the ancestors to make contact. A person is in the wrong job; the ancestors do not want him in that job. But he ignores a thought such as 'I must go and work for Mrs. Smith'P because it does not make sense. This may be an important gift to him. He must show the ancestors that he is willing. He can do a simple thing first, like finding out what type of work Mrs. Smith does. Perhaps he will then write or go and meet her. There are more culprits in the world today because we are losing touch with our own cultures, losing this help from ancestors. We are losing our ability to make spiritual contact." [3]

The Spiritual and the Practical are one

- African Saying

Reentry to my own culture was one of the most difficult transitions I had to make. Though I had lived thirteen years in five countries, adapted to new languages, learned nuances in complex cultures, I still came home with unrealistic expectations. I assumed the transition would be smooth, facilitated by people who spoke my language with whom I shared a common history and background. I did not bring my usual beginner's mind to the situation. My focus was shattered by southern California

---

[3] *Called to Heal*, Susan Schuster Campbell, Lotus Press 2000

freeway traffic and my spiritual communication was full of static.

I wanted to spend more time writing, but struggled to clear my desk of correspondence and administrative tasks. I asked for assistance from God and the ancestors one night before I fell asleep. I asked two simple questions. Should I be writing now? If so, how might I better organize myself? I didn't have a dream that night but woke with a tranquil feeling. I was optimistic that I would find the time to write and that all my tedious tasks would be finished soon.

That same day I noticed that my work went faster. People I needed to contact called me at just the right moment. Unexpected offers were made to help with some clerical work. It all seemed to move easily. The next night I did have a dream. My grandmother Catherine Farrell appeared to me briefly. She held up a stiff piece of cardboard with the number three written boldly on it. She put the number face down and stepped a few paces sideways. She held up the number five. In the dream, I nodded my head, acknowledging I had seen it, again. She put the number face down and showed me the number six. I woke shortly after that.

The next day I remembered the dream clearly but had no clue what "3-5-6" meant. I had a sense that it had to do with my writing but beyond that was uncertain. I let the dream go. I didn't discuss it with anyone. I didn't look for the numbers. This dream had the same texture of many previous dreams in which I received instruction from my grandmother or other loved ones who have passed on. These dreams were always specific and communicated some instruction or information. Eventually, I knew from my experience, the message would unfold.

Several days later, over dinner with my family, my son asked me to tell him a story. Specifically he wanted to know about a conversation I had with a man in Boston. Though the request was odd, I immediately thought of one specific trip. Just back from Africa, we were busy preparing for a move to Poland. During that time, I traveled to Boston to see an old friend. Karin had shared my letters from Swaziland with her new husband, Jim. My letters described my unexpected foray into the lives of African shaman healers. Jim, who understood the publishing business, had sent me a kind note in Africa, encouraging me to write more about my life with the healers.

I remembered that I had taken a few notes during our visit in Boston. I got up from dinner and went to my office in my house. I looked in the file and sure enough, there was an old, raggedy piece of notepaper with some suggestions from Jim. The page started with the advice that I should try writing "three hours a day for five days a week for six months." I cleared my calendar to secure a minimum of "three hours a day, five days a week" and within six months, my first draft of a book was complete.

Now I was on track. However, outside the hours of my writing, I still experienced an overload of filing, correspondence and administrative drudgery. I was thrilled with the help my grandmother had provided on my writing, could she also help with these menial jobs? That night I asked for help again before I slept. In my mind, I asked that God and my ancestors might show me a solution.

That night I dreamt not of my grandmother or other divine guiding spirits, but of my file cabinets and computer. The files in the cabinets were ordered differently. The files in my computer were also reorganized. The dream was very brief but the vision of the reorganization, down to the details of specific names of files, stayed with me.

I could not write without thinking about the files. Finally I set aside a couple days and revamped my files. I labeled each file and folder as instructed, shuffled information, consolidated projects and reorganized papers and diskettes. In the end, the room felt fresh. The process had purged my old work and made room for the new. I actually felt lighter. The chore went surprisingly fast and was relatively painless. I said my thanks to God and my ancestors.

Ancestors and Synchronicity

In the summer of 1999, I was searching for a publisher to buy the North American rights to my book, *Called to Heal*. Ordering from overseas had proved cumbersome and expensive. My overseas publisher contacted potential American firms. There was some interest but whenever negotiations began, problems arose. It was frustrating.

That year the American Booksellers Exposition was to be held in Los Angeles, less than an hour drive from my home. The Book Expo staff expected up to 20,000 people to attend the annual trade show. I narrowed my focus, chose a few smaller networking events to attend and identified the exhibits I would visit. One of the events was a small gathering hosted by the New Alternatives for Publishers, Retailers, and Authors (NAPRA.) NAPRA had promoted the publishing of other works on healing. Perhaps their event would clue me in, help me understand if there was a market for my book.

The evening event was fun and several publishers invited me to visit their booths the next day. It was a thrill to be amongst people so excited about books. I'm not much for cocktail parties and had just about reached my limit. I said my good-byes and turned to head toward the exit when I was introduced to Santosh Krinsky, president of Lotus Press based in Wisconsin.

Forgetting about the pressure to find a home for my book, I was fascinated that this man lived in the state where I had spent my childhood. He explained that Lotus Press was located between Milwaukee and Chicago. My mother came from Milwaukee and my father from Chicago. This was my ancestral land. Santosh had lived in a small southern California city I'd likely not know. He referred to Irvine, where I was then living. Though I was born in southern California, my parents returned to the Midwest when I was five years old. They believed the quality of life was better suited to raising a family. Santosh and his wife returned to the Midwest for the same reason.

I thought this a wonderful conversation to end the night when Santosh said, "Let's see your book. That is a book you're holding there?" Lotus Press proved a champion by staying with a lengthy negotiation and one year later published *Called to Heal* in the U.S. It was truly ancestors driving that meeting and conversation, his, mine and the African healers.

You can't depend on your judgment
when your imagination is out of focus.

– Mark Twain

Ancestral spirits are ever present and available to give you individualized spiritual assistance, if you only ask and listen with your heart open.

They make contact in their own time and in their own manner. Be prepared for constant surprise and little miracles. Albert Einstein said that we could interpret the world in one of two ways. We could believe that nothing that happens in our lives is a miracle or that *everything* that happens is a miracle. He chose the latter, as will you as the joy of ancestral contact increases.

CHAPTER FIVE

Ancestral Dreaming: Messages from Beyond

Ancestors speak to us through our dreams
but we must first prepare ourselves to listen.

– P.H. Mntshali
Swazi Traditional Healer & Zulu Elder

Your "radio" turned on, your ancestors honored, you are now ready for more focused or intentional dreaming with the ancestors. Dreaming can support your exploration into the ancestral collective memory, greater than your own individual history, to draw you closer to living your legacy. The African mystics and healers believe that the ancestors communicate significant information through our dreams. Especially critical are the moments immediately before waking; when we are neither completely asleep nor entirely awake. Your wish, to receive information through your dream states, is perhaps your greatest preparation. Next, you must prepare the body and mind for what the heart and spirit desire.

Cleansing

Five days prior to this dreaming exercise, begin a cleansing process to remove toxins from your system. The cleaner the body, the clearer the dream contact. This cleansing should be gentle and suit your personal practice and methods. Some people use a juice fast for a few days, followed by light meals of vegetables and fruit. Others choose to simply eat less meat that week, substituting fish. Drink plenty of liquids, including a minimum of eight glasses of water a day. Avoid or minimize intake of alcohol, caffeine, tobacco, sugar or other stimulants and/or depressants in this preparation. You will know how best to flush your system of toxins. Again, your willingness, your intent, to be a cleaner, clearer instrument is itself a step toward better contact. In an effort to be this clear vehicle of communication, it is recommended to abstain from sexual relations during the preparation days prior to and the morning immediately after dream contact. This is to clear the energetic fields surrounding you and your body.

Rest and Exercise

Getting sufficient sleep is helpful to good dream recall. Many have told me they have difficulty remembering their dreams. That is not uncommon, especially living in a Western society. We are not trained to pay attention to our dreams. Information from dreams is not understood nor used in our mainstream culture. That can change for you, if you wish.

During this preparation period, try to organize your schedule to allow adequate opportunities to rest. If you need eight hours of sleep, for instance, try to get it. Find peaceful ways to relax and calm your mind. Grab a nap, if you can. This is a great week for a massage, aromatherapy, soothing music, hot baths, and healing fragrances. You'll know just what you need.

Exercise throughout the week. If you have a regular program of exercise such as stretching, walking, running, yoga, Tai Chi, aerobic classes or gym workouts, and can maintain it during your de-toxing without stress, that is fine. If you don't have a regular program, I recommend gentle stretching and walks, especially in nature (city parks, the beach, a tree-lined neighborhood) where you will be a bit further away from pollution, traffic, noise and other distractions. It can be very helpful in calming your body and mind before sleep at night.

Ancestors Leave a Trail

Clues to your own family legacy will be presented in your dreams and eventually during your waking states. As part of the preparation, I urge you to find a moment to consider your lineage. This is a good week to look at old photos of loved ones, hear stories of grandparents and great-grandparents, as far back as there is memory. If you have music that represents your ancestors in feeling or actuality, play it. Allow yourself to be drawn to films, books, colors, and scents. This is a gradual and subtle process. It should not overtake your normal, ordinary routine of daily life. Quite the opposite, it will complement and enhance it.

During this preparation period, you may find yourself wanting to visit or phone family members to chat. These conversations often provide information that reappears in a dream state later. However, it is not necessary to do investigative genealogical work before dreaming. Your preparation should be gentle and come naturally. If you happen to think of someone, call him or her and have a loving talk. Do not put pressure on the thoughts or conversations, simply step back and observe. Notice whom you call and what you discuss. This should be fun and flow easily.

During this preparation, you may be reminded of a family story that has been told repeatedly over the years and handed down through the generations in your family or comparisons made by family such as "You're just like your Aunt Nancy," or "Your Grandpa Johnson would have loved to take that trip." You may find questions popping into your head while listening. Be spontaneous. Ask those questions. They may be just the prompt the person needs to uncover a gem of information.

Intentional dreaming in the African tradition is direct and specific. Scrutinizing the information coming through can actually hinder the flow of contact. I have found this to be true even in this initial preparation stage. Try to stay light in body, spirit, mind, and heart. Don't think too much. Your sense of humor and your willingness are your best allies in this process. Finally, jot down your report to the ancestors; what you are grateful for in your life, what you are challenged by and could use some help with. This is a short exercise, a page or two, focusing on your major gifts and hurdles.

Ready, set, communicate

Dressing in and sleeping on white, natural fabrics is especially good for my own clear dreaming. This is true for many of my African healer colleagues and may be helpful for you as well. If you have had your ancestral party, place the special white cloth under your body or pillow. You may select and light a small fragrance, a candle or incense to further "invite" your ancestors. Certain smells evoke specific ancestors. For instance, Frankincense always invokes my paternal grandmother Catherine. Though we never met in life, she has been active in my dreams for years. Concerning fragrance, I do offer one cautionary tale.

While living in Africa, I had a decision to make concerning two work assignments. I asked for help from my ancestors in my dreams. Before sleep I burned mphepo in a small container on my bedside table. A sage-like, non-hallucinogenic plant, mphepo is the traditional African herb burned prior to making spiritual contact with the ancestors.

Thinking this was an important decision, I foolishly added a bit more dried plant than I would ordinarily. Later that night I awoke to a strong burning smell. The mphepo had continued to burn and filled the room with a light smoke. My husband and I opened all the windows and could not return to sleep until the air had cleared. The healers teased me unmercifully for years after that incident. I should have known better, but that voice which says if a little is good, a lot must be better, was irresistible. I did receive an answer to my question in my dreams and I never burned too much herb again, much to the relief of my family.

Just prior to sleep, slowly relax. If another with whom you sleep distracts you, sleep alone to make initial contact. Even during dreaming, you may feel an impulse to sleep in a different room. Do so.

My African healer friends say that being in relationship with the ancestors, our special angels to the divine, means an endless stream of communication. Step by step, we are led to and through our life's legacy. Though we may have one overlaying "call," daily life still boils down to constant decisions, trials, and opportunities. Your dreaming preparation complete, look back now on the notes you jotted to yourself. Is there a specific question that came up repeatedly during this week?

When asking questions of ancestors, be specific so that the answer is also precise. Let me give you an example. While living in Poland I received a photograph from a client in Ohio. She wanted me to see an image of her recently deceased grandmother. Upon completion of our work, I prepared to return the photo. I could not find it. To make matters worse, I learned this was her only photo of her beloved grandmother and she did not have a negative. Before sleep I formulated the question, "where is the photo?" The next morning I did not remember my dreams but woke with a thought, "the photo is in your office." I looked in my office but it was nowhere to be found. Again I requested help in my sleep. This time I asked, "Where specifically in my office is the photo?" That evening I had a strong dream of my father showing me my desk. The next day, I looked through my desk with a fine-toothed comb, but found no photo.

I did not want to distress my client and was anxious to return her picture. I also knew all things happen for a reason. The timing of the photos return may have been delayed for a reason I could not fathom. I decided to give the search and my dreams a rest. Several weeks later, while Spring-cleaning, I moved my desk away from the wall. There on the backside of the desk, sitting on a small ledge, was the photo. The desk, used in an old Soviet government office, had been built to connect with a co-workers desk. I had never noticed the small lip, which would have attached the two tables.

The client later told me that in her search to replace the photo, she contacted an estranged family member. She was not able to produce a photo, but much healing took place over several long phone calls. Had the photo been in her hands, the client mused, she would have had no excuse to contact this member of her extended family. So, the information did indeed come from my dreams but it was made clear to me only at the exact correct moment, not a minute sooner.

Before sleep, "report" to your ancestors. Refer to the notes you jotted down earlier. Read what you are grateful for in your life, what you are challenged by and could use some help with. Be specific with your request. Ask that a main ancestor identify him/herself to you. Whoever is best suited to give you assistance will come forward. Lastly, as in all things spiritual, ask for only guidance for the highest good. Sleep.

Immediately upon waking, before speaking or interacting with others, write what first comes to mind. It may be a vivid visual recollection. It may be first fleeting thoughts. Do not edit. Do not analyze. Write for about five minutes. What are your first impressions upon waking? What did you see, hear, smell, see or taste during your dreaming? The writing quickly captures the information coming through you. Over time, your observation skills will improve and you may no longer need to actually write the information or your impressions upon waking. I do find that whatever information has been transmitted, will be repeated at the appropriate moment if I forget. The information may be a subtle suggestion, which only reveals itself in its entirety much later; or it may be a direction to be followed immediately, such as my file organizing or Costco trip mentioned earlier. Trust your feelings, you will know the required action, if any, to be taken.

Specifically and generally, through our dreams and waking moments, through all of our senses, we will be contacted. As you wake you may also be reminded of a sound, smell, touch or emotion. We tend to think that we are dreaming only if an image presents itself. Merriam Webster's Dictionary defines a dream as "a series of thoughts, images or emotions incurred during sleep." I am reminded of a radio interview years ago with the famous mythologist, Joseph Campbell. The interviewer suggested that Mr. Campbell's dreams must be quite extraordinary and asked what he "saw" in his dreams. He replied that he saw nothing; rather, he "heard" sounds. Likewise, you may receive information through one sense rather than another. Remember, this is personalized spiritual assistance, designed explicitly to suit you.

We may long for a brilliant dream or dramatic coincidence to prove our dreaming practice successful. You may indeed have such experiences but it is the message, not the "bright lights" of the delivery, which is important. The ancestors and the divine will go to great lengths to capture our attention. However, the incidence of drama wanes as we develop a capacity to understand more and more subtle messages. We ultimately become finely tuned instruments and can receive information and guidance in an ongoing manner. Information is presented and we are privileged to act. Putting one foot in front of the other, we grow braver and more willing to implement guidance and stay in a state of grace.

CHAPTER SIX

Following Ancestral Guidance

The truly great man dwells on what is real,
And not what is on the surface

- Tao Te Ching

A mericans have a penchant for analysis. We scrutinize our intuition and second-guess divine communication. In the corporate world we call it "analysis paralysis." We analyze a situation, document, or deal at such length that pretty soon we are doing nothing. Our contemporary minds do demand empirical evidence to quantify our world. Nonetheless, the limitation of our sophisticated and vital scientific tradition is that it measures only with our five senses. Fortunately we are blessed with a spiritual world beyond the limitations of the physical. The intellect and our contact with this spiritual world form an essential partnership, the perfect balance.

The famous filmmaker Ingmar Bergman once said, "Imagine I throw a spear into the dark. That is my intuition. Then I have to send an expedition into the jungle to find the spear. That is my intellect." Our intellect teamed with our intuition, our ancestral guidance, is relentless and finally successful. With practice we grow confident deciphering and following guidance. Our ability to discern messages strengthens, our integrity is reinforced, our patience grows, and our hearts lead us always toward the greater good for our families and ourselves. However, all this is worth little if we are unwilling to act.

At the conclusion of our 1999 lecture tour, my Zulu colleague and I were asked to see clients as a follow-up to earlier visits. Traditional Healer Mntshali was shocked to learn several clients had not acted on their ancestral guidance, even though communications were now coming in clearly through dream, spontaneous thoughts, as well as incidences of increased synchronicity. He noticed an unusual phrase many used. When asked why they had not moved forward to follow the ancestral instruction, clients often replied, "I am still processing the message." "Aha!" Mntshali said, "Finally, I understand. *Processing* means to 'delay action.' You Americans are funny people, thinking you have all the time in the world. Thinking this life is permanent." Processing life events and relationships most certainly has a place, particularly in personal growth work and therapy, but as we heal our willingness to act on our own spiritual guidance grows ever stronger. Eventually we act even in the face of doubt and discomfort.

You must do the thing you think you cannot do.

– Eleanor Roosevelt

Well into our second frigid winter in Poland, we decided to take a warm weather holiday in southern Africa. My husband had a professional opportunity to explore in Zambia and we added Namibia, Swaziland and South Africa to our four-week itinerary. From Warsaw, it was necessary to connect through South Africa to reach Lusaka, our Zambian destination. As we began our descent to Johannesburg International Airport,

Ron and I both experienced an unusually strong sensation. We looked at each other and almost simultaneously said, "We should work next in South Africa, not Zambia." Even though by this point in our lives we were well experienced in following this inner knowingness, the sheer strength of the sensation was novel. We had one week and a visit to Namibia before we were due in Zambia. Hopefully any action required of us would be made clear.

The time in Namibia was wonderful but a growing feeling toward South Africa distracted us. It became so strong that we agreed to cancel our Zambian sojourn. Our colleague in Lusaka was disappointed but knew us well enough to encourage our "following those feelings." Our visit to South Africa quickly turned from holiday to reconnaissance as our attraction to the country intensified. At last, we surrendered to the pressure and explored schools, housing, and work possibilities. Within months of our return to Warsaw, we were offered a situation that would relocate us to Johannesburg. As it was not the remote Africa we so loved, we might well have resisted the call to this unlikely metropolis. In doing so, we would have unwittingly forfeited an important experience, which deepened our understanding of the country and the region.

Another instance of having to say no involved an uncomfortable action I was guided toward. Over the years, interested filmmakers had approached me with various projects. To date, no collaboration suited the healers or myself perfectly. One team, however, came very close. While living in California, I communicated with the overseas film team for many months. We got to know one another personally and professionally; I believed this partnership could work. Our preparation advanced to the stage where one of the producers would visit the USA to begin some preliminary filming with me. Then the dreams came.

The first dream was simply my maternal grandfather saying, "tell the filmmakers no." This took me by great surprise as I felt the team and I had developed a level of trust well suited to filming sensitive material with the healers. Normally I would have acted on the dream information, but I felt awkward. There was no logical reason and to say no at this point would not be easy. Three days later I had not acted still. That night another dream came. In this dream I was typing on my computer. In the dream I looked up at the screen to read my own words, "I am sorry to inform you that the healers and I are no longer available to participate in the film project." The force of the dream was unmistakable; I must end the project. Several of the healers involved were not accessible by phone. How could I presume to end their participation as well? Nevertheless it was clear that I must.

In the dream I was shown sending a short, impersonal email communication so I took a deep breath and did exactly that. The filmmakers were beside themselves, how could I do such a thing? They were indignant and hurt. In the heat of the disappointment, one of the producers divulged information that proved a serious breach of ethics. Though I was shocked by the indiscretion I was tremendously relieved and grateful that my ancestors had once again provided such perfect guidance. Following the interaction, I posted letters to the remote healers explaining my dream and subsequent action. I later learned that several of the prominent healers were beginning to "feel something was not quite right within the true heart of one of the producers." They were not at all worried, as they completely believed my ancestors would show me how to dissolve the relationship and the project.

Logic and judgment may be reluctant to follow ancestral guidance, especially as we are asked to do unusual things. Initially, we might resist acting but the dream, the thought or suggestion to act recurs. Finally, upon carrying out these instructions, a feeling of well being returns. Often the action results in a direct benefit. After enough of these experiences, we enter a state of grace in which anything from the mere hint of an intuition to a clear and vividly detailed direction from the ancestors is acted upon.

It is only with the heart that one can see rightly,
what is essential is invisible to the eye.

– Antoine de Saint-Exupéry

In the summer of 1997, my family and I were preparing to return home after two years of work in Johannesburg, South Africa. We discussed returning to Washington, D.C. where our personal and professional network was largely based. Shortly after this conversation, I woke from a dream with a strong feeling toward southern California. In the dream, my maternal grandfather who died when I was four years old, pointed to an old friend, Albert, who invited us to relocate near him in San Diego. I had been out of touch with Albert but decided to give him a call since the dream was so strong. He was pleased and *coincidently* had just learned that a long-planned archeological dig in Mexico had been postponed. To his surprise, he would be in town over the summer and offered enthusiastic help.

In the dream I did not hear the specific words, "relocate your family to San Diego." Yet the feeling in my heart to do so was unmistakable. My husband and son concurred, and even though it was not the action we had anticipated, the West Coast did appeal. Then I received an unexpected fax from my mother in Wisconsin. To our surprise, my brother was moving to San Diego to pursue Law School. We had seen Michael only briefly on our rare trips home. We had never lived in the same city, much less the same state. Our son would have an opportunity to know another member of his extended family. This seemed a further verification that we were moving in the right direction. Our travel preparations, actual flights and connections all went smoothly. The maze of logistics necessary to establish a new household unfolded clearly.

The school district we preferred for our son's middle school years was in northern San Diego County. Albert supported his university studies by creating and installing high-end designer wallpaper. He just *happened* to be doing a small job for a client who was a teacher in the preeminent middle school. She was happy to counsel me on the various classes and teachers within the system. I liked her very much but thought it unlikely Joseph would be assigned to her sixth grade homeroom. She taught a special "gifted" class. Joseph's grades were strong but we did not think he needed the added pressure of a high achieving classroom as he re-entered the American school system.

We visited the school and immediately liked the environment. "This is it Mom, this is my new school. I can feel it," he said. The scaled down summer staff was surprised when the very counselor we needed to see popped in unexpectedly to collect some materials for her vacation. The counselor had an impromptu meeting with us and suggested we find a place to live in the attendance area soon. We wanted to rent a house but vacancies were few. The counselor phoned her husband who turned out to be a realtor. He found only one rental home available "but oddly enough," he said, "It is within one mile of the middle school." The house and the school fell into place beautifully.

We wondered what teacher Joseph would be allocated when his information was fed through the computer along with the seven hundred other sixth graders. Remarkably, Joseph was assigned to Albert's client. The chances of that happening had been so slim that it caused us to take a closer look at the special nature of the class and give it a try. Rather than leaving Joseph worried, the teacher taught to Joseph's strengths and creativity. It was in this school that his love for writing poetry first bloomed and later was rewarded with an international award.

The synchronicity was remarkable in all aspects of our new life, professionally and personally. Following the thread from my dream communication, we were each reassured this was the appropriate place to reenter America. The willingness to act, to trust your feelings, to take one small step will usually confirm our interpretation of ancestral communication. One step leads to another and the path is made clear. Do not be afraid to try. If you are stepping in the wrong direction, things will not flow easily and doors will remain closed. Do not worry. The ancestors will show you how to alter your course if necessary.

Mind as Implementation tool of the Heart

If an African has the feeling to carry out an action based on ancestral guidance, she will use her intellect to accomplish that which the heart desires. The mind is seen as the implementation tool of the heart. In American culture, we do not readily receive support for following our hearts. On the contrary, if an action is not immediately logical, we are hard-pressed to explain and rationalize. Therefore, it is imperative that you protect your dreams and ancestral communication from those who do not honor your vision. Overly critical people do not trust their own instincts and are usually not healthy, positive influences in your life.

Ancestral or spiritual communication doesn't always make sense, but it does make a difference. I act when I feel this urge, the ancestral or spiritual urge. It never asks me to do harm, ever. The African master healers believe that harming others diminishes their healing gift and spiritual connection. They have witnessed colleagues who were lured to the dark side by greed or impatience. Even small slips in one's ethical standard will be reflected in weaker concentration and a life that feels less in sync. I have found this to be absolutely true in my own life. Any toxicity, whether it is negative people or unhealthy eating or drinking, can diminish my spiritual contact with the ancestors and God.

Diversion vs. Delay

The African shaman invites us to pause when things are not going as we expect or desire them to. If God and the ancestors are preparing a better-suited circumstance for us, we will be diverted from our original plan. Alternatively, if our next step is not quite ready, we will be delayed until it is fully prepared. The Dalai Lama agrees and says that "when a lot of things start going wrong all at once, it is to protect something big and beautiful that is trying to get itself born. This 'something' needs you to be distracted so that it can be born as perfectly as possible." [4]

Following our move to San Diego, I had a dream in which I heard "You will live in your father's place to complete his dream." I assumed "my father's place" was Chicago. I was nervous to experience the harsh Midwest winters after so many years in warm climates and filed the information very deep in my memory. Chicago didn't ring true for me but I trusted the meaning of the dream would be made clear, if and when I needed to know.

After only one year in San Diego, it became obvious that we needed to move nearer Los Angeles. My husband had joined a firm in Irvine and though he loved the work, the commuter life did not suit us well. I mulled over the move with my mother one evening by phone. A woman who usually worried about our globetrotting and transient lifestyle, she didn't seem bothered by this move. She asked, "What County is Irvine located in?" When I said Orange she told me, "We moved from Wisconsin

---

[4] Pasadena Speakers Program 1999

to California. Had we not returned to be closer to my family, your father's dream was to have a place in Orange County." We moved to Irvine and rented a house. A city of 160,000 people, Irvine was well recognized as a successful planned urban community. Bike and walking paths were abundant, as were lakes and parks. Joseph enjoyed his new school and easily made friends. He aspired to attend the neighborhood Woodbridge High School.

Eventually the time was right to purchase a home. We told our realtor, Sandy that we wanted to keep Joseph in the Woodbridge High attendance area. Sandy suggested the University High School attendance area. Our response was negative. She felt the diverse University neighborhood offered us a lifestyle we were looking for with cultural centers, cafes, a farmer's market and other amenities within walking distance. We said no and persisted with properties in Woodbridge. Much to our chagrin, none of the houses seemed right to any of the three of us.

During this same time, Joseph began to feel strongly about studying Latin in high school. Personally, I loathed taking Latin in high school but Joseph wanted to give it a try. We supported his choice. It was the least we could do given the various languages he had to study over the years including Zulu, siSwati, Afrikaans, French and Polish. Fortunately, Woodbridge High School offered a good Latin program. Of the six public high schools in Irvine, University High was the only other school to offer Latin. The Latin clubs of the two schools often collaborated on events. This sparked Joseph's curiosity and he browsed the University High School web site. Impressed with what he saw, he asked if we might tour the school. While arranging the visit, I learned that it was one of the top ten public high schools in the nation, academically number one in California.

2,000 students broke for lunch as we arrived for our visit. The school bustled but Joseph was not overwhelmed or intimidated. At the office we met our tour guide, Jenny, the Senior Class President. Jenny was lively and honest. She had an uncanny knack for showing Joseph just the right facilities to tweak his interest, the special gardens for earth science classes, the school newspaper office, and the Latin classes. Finally, Jenny looked at Joseph and said, "I hope you do come to school here. It's a great place with good spirit. Whether you do or don't, just remember that high school will be fine, just like the rest of your life, if you can just be yourself." Joseph was dazzled. On the ride home he asked if we could now consider homes in the university area.

Sandy and I started looking the next day. Unfortunately, the townhouses we liked were a bit too expensive. Sandy tried to show me one last unit but had problems gaining entry. The realtor was not available and the lock box didn't open with the normal keys and codes. Peeking through the upper windows on the front door of the townhouse, I could see beautiful Mexican tiled floors. I made a note that the place was very quiet and we should try to see it.

That night, a strange thing happened, our house flooded. An underground pipe from the water heater burst and a gushing leak bubbled up through cracks in the concrete slab. Carpets were torn up throughout the house and it became a disaster area as the repairs and drying out began. Our landlord felt badly about the flood and offered to extricate us from our lease agreement. No sooner had we accepted his offer than Sandy called to tell us we could see the tiled unit. The owner had gotten in touch and offered to show us the unit herself.

The house was lovely, airy and only a fifteen-minute walk to University High School. As much as we enjoyed talking with the owner, the house was still beyond our means. As we left, the owner pulled our agent aside and said, "Ask this nice family to make me an offer." She quickly accepted our reduced offer and worked with us to complete the transaction.

So, Joseph's interest in Latin, our flood, the real estate market, all pointed us to a situation we could not have imagined. We were "diverted" from living in Woodbridge to be placed in a better-suited situation. We were "delayed" from seeing the home we would eventually purchase until such time the owner and we were ready. The dream of my father's was indeed completed with our purchase. We now had "a place in Orange County."

You have likely had experiences that seemed a disappointment or hardship at the time only to find later they were actually a blessing. It takes practice and patience to refrain from instantly judging any situation. With enough experience carrying out ancestral guidance, you will find it difficult to immediately label a direction as good or bad. In time you will simply be happy to have the connection, the contact, the guidance, the relationship of the ancestors.

Once your ancestral connection is initiated or refreshed, you will be given constant opportunities to follow messages that come to you through dreams or capture your attention through a synchronicity of events, or enter your awareness through scent, touch, taste, or touch. Trust your own feeling about the message. Act on what feels right in your heart. Merely act on one thing at a time, placing one foot in front of the other.

Put Ego aside and Serve

Initially, it is natural to race ahead and imagine all kinds of scenarios and even grand results from following ancestral guidance. Over time and with practice, though, we ultimately put aside delusion about the future and are thrilled to simply follow guidance for today. The way in which the future unfolds will surprise and delight you. It will surpass your imagination, if only you can keep your ego in check. An unassuming nature makes a better vehicle for the ancestors. A lesson from my corporate days has helped keep me focused and humble to this day.

I reported directly to the Vice Chairman of a multibillion-dollar bank in Seattle. I gave regular briefings to the executive management committee and the CEO as well. Annually I presented to the Board of Directors. In addition, the nature of my community reinvestment work required many civic meetings and much public speaking. One speaking engagement had me spooked though. The bank president suddenly needed to be out of town and would miss an important commitment. He informed me that the organization would be pleased to have me take his place, especially given this was a tribute to women in business. I was to give a short speech and then introduce the film star Cicely Tyson at a banquet for 1,000 people.

This was a larger audience than I had addressed in the past. The president understood my apprehension and kindly offered me the assistance of his very own speechwriter. I was thrilled beyond belief. Bob was a distinguished consultant to several CEOs who were all excellent speakers. Bob and I had met on a few occasions and I enjoyed his gentle, friendly manner. I was more confident now; sure he would divulge the "special" secrets of dynamic public speaking and all would be well.

The day of our practice session arrived and we met at the majestic Four Seasons Hotel in downtown Seattle. Bob took me to the ballroom and had me stand at the podium, just as I would the next evening. He explained that the larger-than-life television screens on either side of me would broadcast my image and speech to those in the seats at the back of the room. I was terrified; Bob was nonplussed. He had read over my speech and liked the sentiment and stories. Completely relaxed in a seat a few rows back, Bob asked me to give my speech.

I was unnerved by the setting and stumbled on sentence after sentence. I couldn't shake my jumpiness as I imagined the important crowd. I felt horribly inadequate to the task. Bob had me walk around to get the feel for the stage and take some calming deep breaths. Nothing seemed to help. Finally Bob said, "Susan, put your notes down. I want you to think of the audience. Tell me who you think they are." I described accomplished dignitaries and successful business owners. I also knew that there would be some women in the audience who were just starting in business, taking risks of their own. These women would likely have stretched their budgets to attend the expensive event, hoping to glimpse inspiration from those who had already succeeded. Bob jumped up, "That is your audience Susan!" He shouted, "I see it in your eyes. I hear it in your voice. Excellent," he continued, "you have identified your audience and your reason for speaking to them. Now finally I will tell you the most important speaking instruction I give ALL my CEO's."

Bob looked me in the eye and said, *"Put your ego aside, and serve."* He elaborated, "You are an instrument, a communication device if you will. There is something larger than yourself that speaks to all here but especially to your special audience. Think how you can serve them best. Forget about how you look. Yes, yes, yes you'll wear a beautiful outfit and your makeup and hair will be just right, but it is your words coming straight from your heart, which will touch them." The event went well, my speech was a rousing success and I kept my ego in check. The gift to me was the valuable lesson that comes in handy whenever the ancestors contact me with instruction. If necessary, I am willing to appear foolish; to act against current mores, or do whatever is necessary to serve my ancestral guidance.

I implore you then to give up trying to put all the pieces of the puzzle together. Do not even presume it is possible to understand the place a small step has in the future. Concentrate on what is in front of you and give the worry to the ancestors and God. As the African healers say, "We don't have the big picture. The Ancestors do." Be true to yourself and be willing to act. One day you too will find yourself not only comfortable but also eager to remain in the light of this guidance.

CHAPTER SEVEN

Ancestors, a Doorway to the Spiritual

$\mathbf{M}$aintaining this spiritual contact offers a bonus. Not only does it increase our connection to the dead, but also to the living, as I found out. In-between overseas assignments, my family and I were settling into our temporary lodging in Washington, D.C. when I received a remarkable phone call from Jane, a colleague in Swaziland. She had just visited with Grace, a student at the University of Swaziland. Grace and I originally met when she attended my lectures. She was a bright student with a healthy respect for the role ancestors played in her life.

On this day Jane reported that Grace had just arrived in the capital city from her family's village. She had waited five hours on a dusty isolated road for a bus. Semester break was over and she needed to return to classes. Like most of Africa, there were no bus schedules for her region. One simply waited and hoped. Grace explained to Jane, "Finally my bus arrived and Mrs. Campbell was sitting in my favorite seat, just behind and to the left of the driver. I was so surprised to see her that before I realized what was happening, the bus had left without me. I shouted after it but it was too late. There wasn't anything to do but sit down and wait. Lucky for me the next bus came within two hours."

Jane informed Grace that I was not in Swaziland at that time. In fact, I had returned to the United States two weeks earlier. Grace calmly replied, "If so, we must have very strong ancestors. I am sure they had a reason for showing her to me." Sure enough, they later learned that the bus was involved in a serious collision. The passenger sitting in Grace's favorite seat sustained fatal injuries.

Our spiritual connection protects us from harm, as in Grace's case, and alerts us when loved ones need a little extra assistance or attention. Shortly after our arrival in Swaziland in 1991, my husband was called back home to appear at an important trial as an expert witness. A corrupt bank customer stood accused of a large scam, which abused significant loan funds reserved for low-income housing. I decided to stay behind in Africa with our five-year old son. We would be better off staying busy in our new home for the three weeks rather than being so close to what promised to be an intense and grueling court battle.

Joseph and I organized our days to take care of logistics in the morning and enjoy the game parks, markets and cultural attractions in the afternoons. We missed Ron but quickly felt comfortable in this foreign setting. During the last week of Ron's absence, Joseph and I were strolling through a local open-air shopping complex. Leaving the Spar grocery store, we heard a beautiful song played over the intercom system. It stopped us both. I asked a few shoppers if they were familiar with the piece of music. None were. The next day we heard the song again, this time on a local radio station. The title of the song was not announced. Each time we heard it, we both thought immediately of Ron and offered a little prayer for his safety and strength during the difficult trial.

The song continued to follow us. We heard it in another shop, in a friend's car; we even heard a person humming the song in line at the post office. We heard the song for six consecutive days. Finally we learned the music was from an artist named Enya though we still had no title for "our" song and the artist's music was not available in local shops. During this time, Ron and I were temporarily out of communication as our phone and fax service failed; otherwise I would have asked him to try to find the music at home. As the week ended we prepared for Ron's return and forgot about the song, which no longer seemed to be playing.

Reunited in Swaziland, we shared stories of our separate adventures. Ron had brought back a few goodies, current magazines, books and a compact stereo system to replace our little Walkman portables. He told us the story of the successful trial and a particularly exhausting *six-day period* when he was the sole witness being grilled eight hours at a time by the defense attorney. The dates coincided with the days we were unable to reach one another by phone. He said he felt at his very lowest, missing us dearly. He had purchased the CD player and some soft music to help him unwind. There was one CD he was especially fond of as it never failed to make him feel closer to Joseph and I. "I swear I nearly wore it out." he said, "I must have played it every one of those six nights!" He was sure we had not seen this new CD "Watermark" by the artist Enya. He put the CD on and played the one song that soothed him most and called us to his heart more closely. We then heard Joseph's and my "song."

Another time Joseph needed support while I was alone at a movie theater in Johannesburg. It had been a hectic week and I took a break to watch a charming English art film. The beautiful classical soundtrack had me nearly lulled to sleep when I hear the sound of a gunshot. I turned around; the small audience was silently engrossed in the film. There was no violence on the screen. Suddenly, in my mind, I heard my son's voice whisper, "Come home." Though my anxiety may have appeared illogical given the peaceful context, I bolted up and ran to my car. Driving the four blocks home, I felt calmer for having acted, though still on high alert.

As I entered my driveway, my baby-sitter and a young man greeted me. Our usually robust university student seemed weak but relieved to see me. Joseph came from his bedroom to greet me in the living room and the story unfolded. Not five minutes earlier, the babysitter had received a phone call from her parents. Her older sister, suffering from serious clinical depression for some time, had just ended her life. She had taken a gun to her head in her parent's guesthouse in the backyard. The young man, a close family friend, had been dispatched to comfort the sitter as her parents called our house. Joseph had gone to his room, feeling "something was wrong" and said a quiet prayer that I "would come home soon."

Later Joseph and I visited the babysitter and her mother at their home. In the midst of their grief, both offered thanks for the "quick response" when I returned home from the cinema but wondered; how could I have known that I was needed, that there had been an emergency? I shared the story of the "communication." Our hearts ached as the mother hugged Joseph and then spoke of her older daughter, a sensitive soul. We talked of ancestors and her daughters' own ability to reach out as she was passing on, getting my attention. We promised to pray for her reconciliation in God's hands. God and the ancestors work in ways we cannot always fathom. Her daughter, as an ancestor, may one day successfully intervene with a loved one that faces the same fork in the road.

Our spiritual connection also helps us as loved ones make the most important passage, from this life to the next. While living in San Diego, we invited our families to join us for Thanksgiving. Both sides of our families were represented and old friends joined us. My father-in-law, Joe and his wife Marlene, made the drive out from their winter home in Arizona. It was a happy time. Joe seemed unusually quiet that day, happy to sit back in his chair and soak in all the fun and conversation.

Four months later we received a distressed phone call from Marlene. Joe had suffered a heart attack and was in a coma. My husband and his brothers immediately flew to Arizona to be at his side. The doctor's did not give Joe much time. My son and I struggled with whether to stay home or fly to Arizona. Joseph was adjusting to the American school system after years in Africa and was right in the middle of a three-day national testing required for middle school students. Though it would be difficult, I knew we could postpone his test. Something else seemed to hold our feet to the ground.

Though Joe could not speak to us, we believed we could communicate with him. The second evening of my father-in-law's coma, Joseph and I spoke to him from San Diego as my husband held the phone to his ear in Arizona. That evening Joseph was distraught. He remained conflicted about leaving school but felt he should "see Grandpa one more time while he was still in his body." We decided to sleep on it and Joseph dozed off in tears.

The next morning Joseph bounced down the stairs with a big smile on his face and a hug for me. "It's okay Mom," he said. "Grandpa's not even in his body anymore and he's so happy. I saw him in my dream last night and it's okay." I was so relieved to see Joseph happy and relaxed. "But Mom," he continued "Grandpa wants to contact you before he dies." I was flustered and said, "No Joseph, I don't want to hold up Grandpa." Joseph laughed and said, "You know Grandpa. He'll make contact if that's what he wants. You'll see." And he was off to school, feeling resolved about his grandfather.

I said a brief prayer and asked that Joe's passing be blessed and painless. I sent him our love and thanks for all the wonderful memories he was leaving and assured him he would always be in our hearts. I felt very close to him in that moment. Then I sat down to my computer and tried to complete a research paper, which was due for my doctorate program. Appropriately enough, the piece was a study of the Tibetan Book of Living and Dying. Out of the blue I heard Joe's voice say, "Susan, you are a good student. You'll always have time to finish your school work but now I want you to go see a movie." Without thinking I asked, "What movie?" He said, "City of Angels." I hadn't heard of it so I asked, "What is it about?" Joe said, "Impermanence." His voice ended and the room was quiet.

Odd. A career navy man, lover of John Wayne movies, "impermanence" was not a word Joe would have used. Just for fun, I checked the movie listings in the paper. Sure enough, "City of Angels" was playing at a theater down the street. I decided it wouldn't hurt to go to a movie and left my homework for later. The movie starred Meg Ryan and Nicholas Cage, two of my favorite actors. As the film opened, so did my tear ducts. I felt intense sadness at Joe's passing and was thankful to be alone in a dark and fairly empty theater. Gradually I was drawn into the brilliant story. Nicholas Cage plays a benevolent angel who comes gently for people as they are dying. During a failed heart surgery, he witnesses and becomes enamored with Meg Ryan's character, a surgeon. During the devastating surgery, Ryan is able to see the angel of death. Cage's angel makes the difficult decision to give up the beatific life to be with Meg in human form. Powerful scenes of Cage experiencing the simple pleasures of life lifted me completely out of sadness. In the end, though, Ryan's character meets an untimely death and the theme of "impermanence" hits home. I loved the film and walked out silently thanking Joe for this healing gem.

I picked up Joseph from school and we hurried home to telephone Grandpa. It was not to be, Joe had passed away. We called Ron and spoke also with Marlene. I felt moved to tell her my story. She loved hearing of our experience and said, "The City of Angels was the last film Joe saw." I asked what he thought of the somewhat avant-garde film. She said that Joe had walked out of the theater saying, "You know, it wasn't at all what I was expecting." No doubt.

Death and Dying

Psychiatrist Elisabeth Kubler-Ross noted that, in America, we deny death in many ways. We prepare the dead to look as if they were asleep. We often keep our children away from the dying, believing we are protecting them from anxiety or haunting memories. Tibetan Buddhist, Sogyal Rinpoche, says that though death is a vast mystery, it is absolutely certain that we will die, and it is uncertain when or how we will die. Though death is as much a part of living as breathing, Sogyal finds it distressing that the dying remain nearly invisible in Western culture. Ken Wilbur, one of the most influential philosophers of our time, suggests we take our cue from the world of nature where death is not frightening. A very old cat is not consumed with terror or sadness over its imminent death. It calmly walks out to the woods, curls up under a tree, and dies. Such a contrast to the way man faces death.

Unlike Africa where people are born and die amidst community, we remain sheltered. I experienced this sheltering when my father died in 1965. Home unexpectedly from a sales trip, he was experiencing excruciating pain. My mother rushed him to the hospital where he underwent three surgeries. These attempts to save his life failed and within two weeks he passed away. During this time, my brother and I were not allowed to visit my father. Popular thought suggested we two youngest might be scarred with painful memories of my father approaching death. I was disappointed. One day my mother phoned from the hospital. "Bring Susie and Chuck, now," she instructed my older sister. I was excited and hurried to dress. Before we could make it to the door, another call came. We were told not to come; my father had taken a turn for the worse. I lived with regret that I was unable to sit with my father as he passed on. However, many years later, I was given the gift of being with my mother-in-law, Lee, and honored to have held her hand as she breathed her last breath.

Though I had been in frequent dream contact with my deceased father, the experience with Lee provided me extraordinary closure. To be in touch with a loved one as they pass, to experience their spirit leaving the body is an incredible privilege and truly a gift for the living. It intensifies and deeply anchors an understanding that our souls do indeed enter higher dimensions, become ancestors if you will, to remain helpful still. Two days after Lee's death, I experienced her voice speaking to me in my car as I maneuvered Seattle traffic. Her words directed me to a healthier way of life and further cemented my appreciation for the endless connection we have with our loved ones and lineage.

Birth is not a beginning;
Death is not an end.

– Chuang-tzu

Ron felt his mother's light touch at his office. He was back at work a week after his mother's death. It had been a busy and trying period. He felt distracted and struggled to settle into the office routine. Leaning back in his desk chair, he glanced over at the beautiful wooden model boat his mother had presented him on our arrival to Seattle. A beautiful piece of craftsmanship, it also contained a music box. Ron realized he had not wound the music player in many months, distracted by the pressures of work and the very painful passing his mother was experiencing in the last vestiges of cancer. No sooner had the thought crossed his mind than the boat started playing "…and we'll go sailing." It was a lovely reminder of his mother's humor and her sparkle and zest for life.

Several years later, Ron's mother, now his ancestor, brought closure in a more dramatic way. Ron and I were in the early stages of exploring long-term assignments that would take us to Africa as a family. Though we were enthused about the possibilities, Ron worried that his father, now remarried, was perhaps not quite settled enough to face our departure. During this time, Ron woke from a dream late at night and saw Lee sitting at the foot of our bed. Lee told Ron that all was well, that she was very, very happy for our decision to go to Africa. It was to be a wonderful adventure and special time for our family. Joe, Ron's father, also would be well and would share in our enthusiasm. It was now time for all of us to move on. At this, Ron reported, "My mother slowly transformed from opaque to almost transparent. I looked again and she was gone! It was such a spectacular thing, I thought surely you and Joseph would wake but no, you were both sound asleep; the house was completely quiet." From that day Ron, Joseph and I shared an inexplicable sense of comfort and a great exhilaration for our overseas quest. From that point on, things moved more smoothly. Ron's father was very supportive and enthused as Lee predicted. Our adventure took us to Swaziland which proved unique in every aspect, and very "special" as Lee had communicated it would be.

Africans report contact with their ancestors, or those who have passed before them, as natural and easy as speaking with the living. The veil that divides them and us is truly thin, nearly translucent. My sister-in-law in northern rural Wisconsin experienced a beautiful closure when her close friend died with no warning. Her friend was a dedicated police-woman for the sheriff's department, in her early thirties. A single mother of two young children, she had recently married. All who knew them saw a bright future for this special family. Shortly after the wedding Roberta received the call that her friend had died instantly in a car accident. Stunned, Roberta went to bed alone that night, as her husband happened to be working late. Later that night Roberta woke up feeling someone in her room. She saw her deceased friend and heard her say, "I didn't get a chance to say goodbye. I came back to say goodbye. Please don't worry about me. I'm okay." Roberta reported a reconciled and calm feeling afterwards. Indeed, it felt, her friend was "well taken care of and at peace."

My cousin Jerry Synold, inducted into the Hall of Fame by the California Association of Alcohol and Drug Abuse Counselors for his pioneering work with the US Navy, was only seventeen years old when my father died. Years later, Jerry shared an encounter that took place several days after my father's passing. Angry and heartbroken at the loss of his favorite uncle, Jerry wanted to only "keep moving to numb the pain." Hitchhiking out of Milwaukee, Wisconsin Jerry reported feeling angry and wondered what kind of God would take such a man, so full of life and laughter? Jerry stood on the side of the highway, waiting for another ride that would take him further and further away from home and the reality of his uncle's absence. No ride was forthcoming and for some time he stood alone. All of a sudden he felt my father's presence and a hand touched his shoulder. He heard my father's voice tell him that all was as it should be, that he was fine. "You do not have to be angry any longer," my father comforted him, "Return home, live your life and keep your heart open." Jerry said that "an incredible feeling" came over him and he felt not only an "amazing tranquility" but also a resolve to be as vivacious in following his dreams as his Uncle Jack had been.

On one of my African excursions I drove my Landrover to an isolated African village to meet with a healer who was also a headmaster of a regional boarding school. An African colleague accompanied me to navigate and make the introduction on arrival. As we neared the healer's village I noticed a slow sad procession of high school-aged students led by an older gentleman. "That is him," Moses my companion shouted. "Pull over and let us say hello." It was a funeral procession we were observing and the gentleman was the healer we were hoping to meet. Thinking this was a distressing and inopportune day to visit, I was greatly surprised by the smiling face of the healer when he realized we were his visitors. I offered condolences as we learned his student had been killed in a car accident. The healer said, "This is not a sad day. My student, Faith, will be a tremendous help to us, as she becomes an ancestor. We are so very lucky to have had her with us as long as we did. She was our gift from the ancestors. No, we must not be sad for we want her to move forward and do this powerful work with the ancestors."

The ancestors also provide a phenomenal source of protection in precarious moments. My family experienced this incredible safety shield in an extremely dangerous situation overseas. It happened during our assignment in Johannesburg, South Africa.

It was a typical Saturday morning. Joseph and I lounged around the house in our pajamas while Ron prepared for a breakfast meeting with a visiting colleague. Joseph sat in front of our new television hutch, sorting his videos on the bottom shelf. Suddenly his face lit up with a big smile as he said, "Mom, I've got a great idea! Let's have a breakfast meeting of our own. We don't have to go far. We can just walk down the street." I liked the idea, too.

Ron left for his meeting while Joseph and I walked up the street to our favorite little café run by a British family. It was a beautiful, sunny day with the normal morning noise. Gardeners and cleaning staff worked a half-day on Saturdays so the mood was playful as Africans called out to each other across the lawns and sang loudly. We heard dogs barking, children playing outside, we waved to neighbors. Nothing was out of the ordinary.

We enjoyed our breakfast and started a lazy stroll home. When we were two blocks from our house though, Joseph and I both noticed something extraordinary. There was no noise. We heard no birds chirping, no dogs barking, no people talking. In fact, there were no people. We saw no one in the vicinity. Joseph commented at the time that it felt like a "shield or bubble" was over us. It did seem surreal, like a Twilight Zone episode where we were transplanted to a different dimension sans life forms. We were so relaxed, we even joked about the strangeness. We felt no fear or danger of any kind until I reached our kitchen door and I heard my deceased father's voice say, "Open the door but keep Joseph at your back."

I tucked Joseph behind me, held his hand firmly and slowly opened the door. The house was in a shambles. I looked up and saw armed men fleeing through my backyard. I closed the door, took Joseph's hand and walked away from the house, in the opposite direction. It took only seconds. I called Ron on my cell phone and we alerted our security company. Our neighborhood soon swarmed with guards and police.

To gain access, the thieves not only used an axe to chop down our heavy oak side door but also sliced it into kindling. Windows were smashed and the house ransacked. Oddly enough the robbers left behind piles of goods they had organized to take with them, suitcases half-packed with our clothes, blankets with electronic devices stacked in the middle. We were perplexed. The design of our house and the way it was situated on our lot would have prevented the robbers from actually seeing us approach. Even if they heard us coming near, it would not have allowed sufficient time to run as far as they did.

The police were stunned. What caused these brutal thieves to run away? Why had they not shot us and finished the job? They could easily have overtaken a woman and a small boy. Violent crime was on the increase, they told us, and this was the more typical scenario. What or who spared our lives that day? The burglars were never found. Our goods were never returned. In my statement to the authorities I told of the bizarre absence of sound and people. Afterwards the police were very solemn as they told my family that we "were incredibly well protected by the ancestors." My family and I could not have agreed more.

CHAPTER EIGHT

Legacies: Gift of the Ancestors

Throw away the idea that people die... Ancestors do good and
powerful work. Because they did not complete their assignment in their own lives, they have work to do now. You
cannot weigh your own life. The ancestors come to give you a
legacy; they know what is the best life for you. They are
serving you. You may think you know better but you cannot
have all the information, only the ancestors
can see the whole picture.

– P.H. Mntshali, Swazi Healer & Zulu Elder

Encarta World Dictionary defines
legacy as "something that is handed down or remains from a previous
generation or time." We each carry the seeds of ancestral legacies; the
unfinished work, undeveloped talent, incomplete travel, unhealed family
wounds and other important vestiges of those who have gone before us.

Whether we are cognizant of our lineage or not, ancestral gifts will be presented. It is often in retrospect we see the impact of their connection.

Rob was a successful California executive in the computer industry when he attended my lecture on ancestral communication. He had a love for Hawaii and mentioned his desire to visit more often; perhaps even travel further into the South Pacific. Rob's wife noted that his study at home was decorated with artifacts from Bali, though they'd never been to visit.

An only child, Rob's parents and grandparents had passed away early, leaving precious little information about his ancestry. He glanced through a box of unsorted black and white photographs he had inherited. There were few clues. One photo did show a large house and noted the town in Maine where his father had been born. Growing up, he had heard few stories about Maine. There were no trips back to visit family.

An invitation to attend a convention in Boston got Rob looking at maps. He could take a few more days off and drive up to Maine. Armed only with the photo, Rob headed toward his father's home. He stopped to speak with the post office manager, chatted to locals in the cafes. One contact led to another. He eventually found the very house in the photograph and met an elderly couple that had actually known his father and grandfather. He was greeted warmly and treated to many old stories of his family. One story in particular hit close to home. Yes, Rob's grandfather did move the family west and settled in California, where Rob was eventually born. However, his grandfather's dream was not to settle in California, but to move further, to explore the South Pacific. The shamans would say that unable to fulfill the dream, the grandfather now passed the legacy to Rob.

Negative Fixation flip side of Positive Passion

Africa has long called my husband and I, though in the beginning, it presented itself in opposite emotions. In 1976 I applied from my home in Madison, Wisconsin to serve as a Peace Corps Volunteer. The process was comprehensive and moved at a snail's pace. Finally my application was accepted and the Peace Corps staff in Washington, D.C. discussed regions of the world I might serve. I was interested in nearly all parts of the world, but not Africa.

I remember the staff person's surprise. "Not Africa, why? It's an incredible continent! Are you sure?" I didn't understand the strong feeling myself but I said no, I was not ready for Africa. It seemed a very mysterious continent, culturally too exotic. This was not a rational synopsis given the other countries I was willing to consider. Still, my negative feeling toward Africa remained strong. After months of reviewing assignments, I was drawn to the Solomon Islands. The last person in my family to have been in the South Pacific was my father who served with the Navy in Guam during World War II.

At the same time, my future husband Ron was applying to the Peace Corps from his home in Oregon. When the recruiter asked for his geographic preferences he said, "I want to go only to Africa." His was an equally powerful though opposite feeling. Regrettably, the jobs available did not match his skills and professional interests very well. He was disappointed each time he had to turn down an African assignment. It was maddening. Eventually a job in the Solomon Islands seemed strangely perfect. Ron's father and uncle both were excited for Ron as they remembered the beautiful terrain of the Solomon Islands when their Navy ships stopped in Guadalcanal.

In the Solomon Islands Ron and I found not only a profound love for each other, but also a growing mutual passion for international work. Funny enough, our first overseas assignment as a married couple sent us to Africa. My apprehensions about the region had dissipated. The African healers say my initial negative response to Africa was divine intervention by the ancestors to prevent my traveling ahead of time. They believe, as do I, that our individual legacies of travel to Africa were linked. It was significant that we be united when we first stepped foot onto the continent. Such was the way of the ancestors, approving our union and blessing our call to Africa.

We departed for a two-year project in Botswana just three weeks after our wedding. Africa thoroughly seduced us. Not only were we fascinated by work with the various tribes and governments, but also the land itself seemed oddly familiar though neither of us had ever lived in such desert landscape. Eventually, our own son would share a deep passion for the continent, especially the southern region. Nonetheless, these connections, my professional focus on spiritual work of the ancestors, and our twenty-year relationship with Africa had failed to produce any physical sign, not even a trace, of our own forefathers having been to this continent.

You might think at this point that a bit of genealogy research would have been useful? I did investigate but found no traces of an ancestor who had made it to Africa, much less this specific southern section. I must admit though, my desire to make advanced inquiries was minimal at best. The phenomenon of comfort and familiarity I consistently experienced in Africa was so complete that delving further into our family trees felt irrelevant. What would it show me? That I had ancestors who had come to Africa? I could sense that was the case. It was only when I was at home in America, back in a linear, logical culture that I would wonder.

The thread unravels, signs of family in Africa

Back in California, my then twelve-year-old son woke from a dream. Still a bit drowsy, Joseph described being in an underground mine of some sort. "A European man, an ancestor, worked there," Joseph reported, "He wants some flowers at my window." Joseph picked some small white flowers from our garden and placed them at his windowsill, said a little prayer for this ancestor and headed out to play. Ron vaguely remembered an ancestor named Chapman Thompson who had come to America as a boy of five. Chapman's parents died before he was seven. At the age of ten, the story went, he had started working in the mines, perhaps he was reaching out to Joseph.

Fast-forward three years as Joseph discussed the upcoming Career Day at his high school. He named the university representatives that would be available to discuss their programs. We were excited; the prospects for his interests were numerous. Yet, for a child who has talked about university since he was in elementary school, he seemed strangely indifferent. When pressed, he said, "Well, all of these universities are in America. What if I don't go to a campus here? Maybe I will go to university in Scotland!"

Scotland? This was news to us but clearly Joseph was captivated. "Any university in particular?" we asked. Without skipping a beat, Joseph said, "I've been checking out websites for universities in Scotland. The

University of Edinburgh looks great to me." Evidently this was no frivolous notion. We offered to help Joseph explore the possibilities. Ron remembered a Scottish colleague, a university professor he had worked with some years back. He promised to speak with him.

The Scottish colleague was not in Ron's address file so he looked through a couple storage boxes in our garage. Sifting through files and documents, he stumbled onto papers my father-in-law had left for us. Amongst them was an obituary from 1920 for his ancestor Chapman Thompson, who the clipping noted, was actually *Joseph* Chapman Thompson. So it was no surprise after all that he had made contact with our son, his namesake. He read further, "An eager ambition led Thompson to improve himself in spare moments of study. He paid particular attention to mining and, in time, graduated as a Mining Engineer from Rutherford College at Newcastle-on-Tyne. Later he was recognized for his contributions in mining research at the *University of Edinburgh, Scotland.* His superior skill secured for him positions of importance in the mining fields of the United Kingdom."

Eventually he returned to America where the Governor of Illinois called him "singularly successful" as the Director of Mines and Minerals in that state. The obituary ended, "His life stands forth as a remarkable illustration of human possibilities." Like his ancestor Thompson, our son Joseph had left his own country, America, to live overseas at age five. That we took Joseph to live in the southern region of Africa, the well known *mining region* was no doubt well appreciated, if not orchestrated, by the ancestor Chapman himself.

As these revelations of our lineage were unfolding, I was off to Africa on business. I included a stopover in Swaziland to visit my mentor, P.H. Mntshali. We sat on the floor of his mud hut and pondered our unlikely friendship, a traditional African elder of prominence and an American middle-aged white woman. We marveled at the wonderful magic behind our alliance. As I was preparing to leave, P.H. said, "Oh, Dear Me, girl! I almost forgot to tell you. I am getting to be an old man! Look, it is this trip you will see a sign of your ancestors in Africa. My ancestors are in communication with your ancestors. They advise it will happen before you depart for America. Don't worry my dear. It is enough that you have a relationship with Africa. That is your legacy, pure and simple." He laughed and hugged me good-bye. I had not a clue of what the "sign" would be.

Cape Town was my next stop, the most European of the southern African cities. Surrounded by the ocean, the magnificent Table Mountain and the gorgeous vineyards of the wine country, it is a world-class center. As stunning as it is, I did not warm immediately to Cape Town twenty years ago. My heart and soul were more at home in the remote, dusty areas of the region. I felt disconnected from "my" Africa in this European bastion. However, when my research with African healers expanded to include the low-income townships surrounding the grand city, I began to appreciate the diverse population and complexities of Cape Town. I was looking forward to this visit, my last stop before my return home.

Business in Cape Town kept me busy for a week. One colleague suggested a drive around the Cape of Good Hope. We would be able to discuss our project as well as enjoy the ambiance of the small fishing towns on the route. Splendid idea, I organized my notes and materials and headed out for a day of fun. We were driving south of the city, hugging the dramatic coastal drive when my associate pointed out Chapman's Bay and Chapman's Peak, the imposing mountain guarding the water. I was astonished. So this was the "sign" P.H. had alluded to. I could easily picture Ron's ancestors arriving from Scotland and England; recuperating from the grueling journey in this lush, green oasis before heading north to the vast openness of the plains. Facing an uncertain new start in a wild and hostile environment must have been daunting. I was tremendously moved. I honored and silently thanked them for clearing the way for us, their modern progeny.

We continued round the Cape, stopping at scenic villages for lunch and later tea. Completely satiated with the beauty around us, the wonderful food and the ease with which our work concluded, I nearly missed another ancestral sign. Heading back to Cape Town, nearly parallel to the Chapman Bay on the western side of the Cape, was none other than *Schuster Bay*. Like a wink from the ancestors, I was shown a dramatic trace of my own father's ancestors, the Schuster's. A further "sign," it confirmed what my heart already knew. My husbands' ancestors and mine had been working together and our legacies were indeed well linked.

What's in a name?

One family found an extraordinary healing legacy in a name nearly lost. Home from college for the weekend, Sasha told her parents of a pervasive desire to change her last name. She and her parents were close and had always been able to talk through any problem, until this. "I don't understand. Why would you want to drop our family name? Change it? Change it to what?" asked her mother. Sasha told them a remarkable story.

Earlier in the year she had woken from a dream. She remembered no details, only one word, the name "Dean." This was peculiar as she knew no friends, no teachers, no relatives with this name. Several weeks later, she had the thought; "I should change my name to Dean." Where did that come from, she wondered? She could make no sense of it yet it felt a superb idea. Whenever she thought of her name as Sasha Dean, it seemed even more natural than her "real" or given name. The idea persisted, coming to mind several times throughout each day. Eventually she actually looked into the legal procedure for changing her name in her local court system. It was time, she decided, to tell her parents.

There was no denying that Sasha's desire to change her name was quite serious and that it seemed to give her not only joy but also a certain calmness her parents had not seen before. After the weekend together, they gave their blessing and Sasha proceeded to change her surname to Dean. Sasha's mother was scheduled to visit her own mother and grandmother later that week. Though the name change did not seem as bizarre in fact as it had in theory, she was nervous about sharing the information. She trusted just the right moment would present itself and the perfect words would come to mind. She loved her daughter and her mother; it was not a conflict.

As it turned out, that perfect moment came fairly soon after the three women sat down to coffee. Sasha's mother got as far as mentioning the name Dean when her grandmother began to tear-up, and a long hidden family story emerged. A young woman, several generations back on the grandmothers' family, had become pregnant out of wedlock. Her family was of a high social standing in their city. Having a baby outside marriage would be considered a great disgrace. The family banished her to a distant convent where she discreetly had the baby. However, rather than give up the baby for adoption as agreed, she decided to keep and raise the child on her own. Not wishing to disgrace her family further, she vowed never to return home. Before leaving the convent she sent word to her parents of her decision and informed them that she had taken a new name to further disguise her lineage. He new surname would be Dean, her father's first name.

This story had been hidden for many years. The grandmother had learned of it when she was just a child. She overheard her own grandmother telling the story and begged that it never be told again, for the sake of their "good name." Sasha's grandmother took this as a severe warning and never repeated the story to a soul. The extended family later held a short ceremony in the form of a prayer service at their church to honor this Ancestor Dean and welcome her back into their family's heart. From all accounts, it was a genuinely moving and healing event.

Legacy calls attention through Illness

The ancestors are believed to reach us through a continuum of contacts. First a subtle suggestion, then further gentle coaxing followed by a stronger "push," such as an idea you simply cannot get out of your head. Finally, serious illness is a "last ditch attempt" to capture our attention. We may first be contacted through any or all of our senses, dreams, synchronicity, and intuition. If these all prove unsuccessful and we resist the divine benevolent direction, we may begin to suffer physical unease and ultimately illness. In some cases the specific nature of the ailment may itself be a clue to a long festering wound in an ancestry, such as the woman with symptoms mimicking a palsy in her hands and arms.

A businesswoman approached P.H. Mntshali and I following our lecture in Washington, D.C. She was in obvious distress and complained of a mysterious malady. We witnessed her hands shaking as she spoke. For the past year the woman had experienced symptoms of a degenerative disorder. It was increasingly difficult, she said, to use her hands for the most ordinary tasks. The quivering that had started in her hands became stronger and was now moving into her arms as well. A well-educated woman, she researched her situation and underwent a battery of medical tests but her doctors could find no physical evidence of actual disintegration that might have caused this trembling. She experimented with diet, exercise, and meditation. Nothing helped. The shaking continued.

P.H. and I stated the obvious. Since she had been drawn to our lecture, there might be some ancestral connection with her physical ailment. We suggested she have her own ancestor party and do the dream exercises, the same simple steps outlined in this book. We left a contact number for her to follow-up on our return to the West Coast. P.H. and I had seen this shaking in clients before, in Africa and in the U.S.A. In some cases it mimicked a variety of behaviors of an ancestor in an act that had been unresolved through the lineage. Several weeks later the woman phoned with a report. She had followed the straightforward instruction and though she had no specific dreams she did have a memorable visit with a relative the next week.

A favorite aunt had met her for dinner in Old Town Alexandria, Virginia. Now a charming colonial tourist venue, Alexandria had once been one of the nation's principal ports. Two hundred years ago, its strategic location on the Potomac River made it a bustling center for exports. The aunt said the place reminded her of an old family rumor about an ancestor who allegedly killed a woman and fled the country from this very port. A colorful myth perhaps but a good story all the same.

The young man, the story went, had fallen on hard times and was in the port town struggling to make a living. In a desperate moment, he jumped out at a woman in an alleyway, hoping to snatch her purse and run. "The woman dropped her handbag but was so frightened that she began screaming and our ancestor supposedly panicked and killed her, running off with her handbag," the aunt understood. "I can just imagine," she continued, "if it had been me, I would have been trembling, too." And at this she demonstrated by shaking her hands, then her arms, until her entire upper body was trembling. "Suddenly my aunt stopped and apologized for telling such a story given my own battle with shaking symptoms. 'No,' I said, 'Quite the contrary. I think you've given me a clue!'"

The woman told her aunt of the ancestor party and together they decided to offer homage to the murdered woman's family. They gave a short prayer before dinner, asking for forgiveness and healing between the two families linked by this brutal act. Last I heard from the woman, she was feeling much better. Her shaking had not subsided but was occurring less frequently. She said she was still exploring a medical solution to her symptoms but also researching the ancestral story. She suspected there were other clues to help reconcile the injustice that had come to her attention. Though unexpected, this "legacy" had provided some relief. She was feeling optimistic about the prognosis for her condition.

A professional Calling passed through Legacy

A legacy can also present itself as a calling to specific life work. Imagine a family has a legacy for architecture. The call to building design first comes to the grandmother. As a child she constantly "builds" structures with sticks and blocks. During family trips to downtown Chicago, she demonstrates an insatiable appetite for visiting the tall buildings so foreign to her rural existence. However, her interest in architecture is stifled in high school. The times offer no such trade for a proper young woman. Though frustrated by the closed doors that meet her passion, she is comforted by her new love for a young banker. They marry and move to the city. Here at least, she enjoys raising their children in the shadows of the beautiful buildings and teaches them to appreciate building design. She ends her days with a bit of melancholy, wondering what it would have been like to develop her own interest in architecture.

Next, the ancestors try her son. The grandmother, noticing his particular interest in building, had provided opportunities to further stimulate his curiosity. As an adolescent, he delights in outings to building sites and willingly joins his mother on architectural tours. He is about to pursue architecture at university when he is drafted into the army during World War II. His talent and young life end on the battlefield in France. At this point, the ancestors become frustrated. No one yet has been the perfect vessel for this inheritance. A generation is skipped. The interest in architecture is lost. Not mentioned at family gatherings, no vestige of this latent family talent remains.

Unaware of this legacy, the grandson begins to notice that his small daughter loves to construct things with her play toys and blocks. She shines in math and sciences. Her teachers mention an uncanny eye for detail and enthusiasm for drawing complicated structures. She even gives up a friend's birthday party to help her father with a kitchen remodel, preferring to "build" rather than play. The seed of the ancestral legacy has been planted. She is possessed of the talent, blessed with the gift. Though the grandson lives in Arizona, the girl, a young woman now, is drawn to the Midwest where she attends the University of Chicago. She excels in architecture. Her gift grows and she works with it late into her old age, even teaching long after she retires as partner of her architectural firm. Now the ancestors are pleased. A legacy, a thing of loveliness has been passed on. An inheritance restored, an ancestor's dream, fulfilled.

The light which departed souls radiate is responsible
for the progress of the world and the advancement
of its peoples. They provide the supreme moving impulse
in the world of being.

– Gleaned from the writings of Baha'u'llah
Baha'i Faith

Ancestors are compassionate and generous beings with the best interest of their descendants at heart. Their own advancement in the spiritual dimension depends upon the completion of unfinished business, which may be the gift of an undeveloped talent or making amends for callous acts or deeds committed during their lifetime. The ancestors' capacity to pass healing gifts and grace their progeny is boundless. Whether we are cognizant of our lineage or not, these ancestral gifts will be presented and your true calling will unfold.

CHAPTER NINE

Callings and Unclaimed Gifts

A calling can come at any stage of life. An impulse to follow a particular career or a strong urge to do a particular type of work beckons young and old alike. More than a single talent or profession, a calling is a way of life. Once acknowledged and activated, or merely glimpsed and imagined, the call leaves us dissatisfied with alternatives of less substance or challenge. The call is higher than reason, urging us on when we feel we have no road map.

If we deviate from our call's path, we return time and again until finally we give ourselves fully. We eventually look back and wonder how we could have lived otherwise. I have found that no matter the culture, we all seem to know, at a deep level, when we are not following our call. We are unhappy. We are restless. We feel increasingly uncomfortable with our work. We must move on without judgment, be grateful for this work, appreciate the lessons we may have learned and pray for guidance that we might seek out our true calling. We honor our ancestors, our spiritual connection. What we must do, will be shown to us at the right time.

I have seen very talented people become sidetracked or distracted by commerce, or the business of making their "calling" provide an income to meet their expectation. As for financial security, let me quote the African healers, "it all depends on how you obey orders. If you obey exactly as the ancestors direct, your practice, your life, will not fail. The ancestors will provide. They will show you a way. At first you may worry. How will you pay your bills, the children's' school fees? Then you become caught up in your calling, your true work, and your love for it grows. Soon you are only serving and not worrying so much about the bills. When you need it most, money or goods arrive. Your calling is God's work. God does not call us then leave us to drown in hardship."[5]

Every man dies.
Not every man truly lives.

– Braveheart

A calling is not a light obsession, it's not something that sort of feels like I want to do this or I could walk away from it. I believe there is no walking away from a calling, if you want to truly live a full life. The call links us to our past and sheds light on our future. It is unavoidable, exists for the greater good, heals within our ancestry and prompts us to fulfill our deepest dreams. Once accepting or acknowledging a call, we are naturally drawn to adjust our work or personal lives accordingly. Steps are made clear and help is provided as we attract appropriate people and circumstances into our lives. We may not understand the full implications of these otherworldly impulses but, if we are willing, we will be directed in spite of our own inadequacies. Mother Teresa is an extraordinary case in point.

An Albanian from Yugoslavia, Mother Teresa came from peasant stock, from a community of hill people. Though not well educated or trained, she was completely subservient to God, obeying intuitive promptings and spiritual direction without questioning. As she explained

---

[5] *Called to Heal,* Susan Schuster Campbell, Lotus Press 2000

in an interview in the 1980's, "God's 'call' came to me...the message was quite clear, I was to leave my convent and work with the poor while living amongst them. I knew where I belonged but I didn't know how to get there." She moved forward with such complete trust that nothing was impossible. The action she was to take unfolded gradually, as is the case with a calling.

Our mission becomes more obvious over time, one step at a time. The general message and divine direction is often clear but the specific details may have to slowly present themselves. Our experience soon teaches us to trust these promptings. Our risk "muscle" strengthens and we grow willing to take greater and greater risks to serve the calling. As we gain experience we will be both supported and challenged. It becomes increasingly important to keep balance in one's life, to honor your integrity and to live an ethical life. If so, clearer guidance in both our sleeping and waking hours will follow. My African colleagues used to say, "Susan, if a person is not one hundred percent for you, they are against you. Leave them or they will drain your courage to follow your dreams." Initially I thought this harsh guidance. Over the years, though, it has proven of the utmost help. It has saved me time, effort, resources and poorly matched friendships and business relationships.

"The ultimate measure of a man is not where he stands in moments of comfort and convenience, but where he stands at times of challenge and controversy."

– Martin Luther King, Jr.

A true calling will not allow you to merely "sit on the fence," vacillating between full-blown dedication and passing interest. At some point you will face a juncture, a moment of reckoning. In my early work with the African healers in Swaziland, I faced pointed criticism from colleagues who were certain I was committing professional suicide. Rejecting lucrative management consulting contracts in order to spend more time with traditional elders and mystics seemed ludicrous to many. There were moments when I, too, wondered about the viability of my ever-growing interest. The World Bank and the King of Swaziland were to figure prominently as I faced the juncture of my own calling.

While still juggling consulting work with research on the African healers, I eagerly awaited a short-term assignment with a World Bank team headed to Zimbabwe. This was a project I had been interested in for years, a new approach to small business lending that I had long advocated. As the only woman and the only American on the assessment team, this was a feather in my cap. Some logistical and contractual issues delayed the team's start date so I continued with my scheduled visits to the healers. The bureaucratic process bogged down further causing additional delays. Finally, the anticipated call came from Washington, D.C.; I was to join the team the following week. At the same time I received an invitation to meet a distinguished African healer; an invitation I had been hoping to receive for the past six months. The date I was to meet him *happened* to be on the same day I was to start the project for the World Bank. In my heart I knew what I must do.

I called Catherine, my World Bank contact, and told her I could not accept this coveted assignment. When I explained why, Catherine said, "You are certainly aware Susan, that you have just crossed the line. Your work with the healers has ceased being a hobby." It was startling, but true. She wished me luck as word traveled swiftly throughout my professional network. Many shook their heads and called me truly mad.

My husband and I were unsure how my decision would affect his own work. As a World Bank advisor to the Government of Swaziland, Ron had a public profile. He was quoted in newspapers, interviewed on radio and television. What, we wondered, would the Cabinet Members and even the King think of my forays into African traditional spirituality? Would Ron be considered less credible for my having such close contact with the healers? Would his advise be mistakenly linked to African mystics? How much of a liability was my new calling? We didn't have to wait long for the answer.

Ron was soon called to the palace to give a briefing to the King. At the conclusion of the briefing the King turned to Ron and said, "I understand your wife is working with the traditional healers." Ron hesitated, uncertain how my unusual contact would be received. The King removed any doubt as he told Ron that he was well aware of my good standing with the elders and very pleased with the research I was doing. He also knew that prior to my arrival, the healers reported premonitions and ancestral dreams that conveyed the significant relationship I would build with them. He shook Ron's hand and praised our family. With the King's blessing, my decision to devote myself to my calling, to my unexpected work with indigenous spirituality, was sealed.

No one can make you feel inferior without your consent.

– Eleanor Roosevelt

Our feelings are another access point for the ancestors to communicate with us. If you have doubts about a friend, colleague or loved one, observe closely how you feel when with them. Are you exhausted when ending a phone conversation with them or energized and recommitted to your own path? Acknowledge and honor your true feelings. They are precise signals. Steer clear of individuals and groups who leave you feeling confused or deflated. I have found over the years that those who would say our yearnings don't make sense, are illogical or unrealistic are best given a wide berth. These individuals have their own calls in life, their own paths to follow. Let them go their own way or as Voltaire said, "Think for yourself and let others enjoy the privilege of doing so too." Protect and nourish your calling. Those who love us, whether they understand our calling or not, will support us in our efforts. True love and caring can do no less.

Another piece of African advice I treasure is "Put no pressure on your call and the ancestors." In our culture, we have grown to expect immediate gratification and are anxious to understand the future. With ancestral legacies and callings, this is not always possible or desirable. Dr. Jane Goodall, in exploring her own spiritual odyssey said of her lecture responsibilities, which grew exponentially in her later years, that if she had known at that time that her efforts would keep her more or less permanently traveling, she might not have been strong enough, committed enough, to start out along such a hard road.

We can implore but not demand God and the ancestors to provide us earthly benchmarks. However, our culture will still demand an explanation when our "progress" does not match their expectations. Let me illustrate. A couple years ago I was flying to South Africa to launch *Called to Heal*. I looked forward to the promotion of my first book. I was impressed with the marketing plan and itinerary of events my publisher had organized. My book was assured prominent display in the major bookstores; my guest appearances were on popular shows. On my arrival, though, my heart sank as my publisher explained an "unfortunate mistake." Instead of their marketing department releasing only my book in October as planned, a best-selling South African novelist's latest offering was sent to all the retailers as well. The stores with limited space chose to use my display space for the new hot novel. I could hardly blame them. This guy was a sure bet and his latest book looked enticing. I was disappointed yet some greater feeling suggested it was not a failure.

My interviews went well while my book remained practically invisible in the shops. Nonetheless, audiences called into the shows wanting to discuss *Called to Heal*. I was so pleased that anyone had actually found the book, let alone bought and read it, that I thanked each caller on air. All creative projects have their own life force and this one was showing me to whom it was delivering its message. The feedback was very personal and insightful. Laborers and housewives, students and professionals were finding the book useful.

At the end of my three-week tour, I made plans to travel to Swaziland to greet my colleagues, especially P.H. Mntshali. I returned to Johannesburg from Cape Town and packed for the road trip to remote Siteki, near the Mozambique border. I had completed my promotion obligations and looked forward to some relaxation. I collected phone messages and returned a few calls. The calls were remarkable. A janitor at a broadcasting company mentioned *Called to Heal* to a secretary. Surprised equally by his literacy and his willingness to spend hard earned cash on a book, she told her boss, an assistant producer. The assistant read the book and presented it to executive producers.

While this was going on, I returned a call to my publicist who informed me that she had failed in her pitch to the country's most popular news magazine television show. The program did not promote books.

In fact, in ten years they had highlighted only one. I thanked her for her effort not realizing that my last call was from the very same network program. What the well-connected publicist could not accomplish, a janitor had. I was soon traveling with a news crew and introducing them to my book, the second to be promoted on their show in ten years.

Take the long view before judging any single event a success or failure. All experiences are simply part of a larger picture, a larger plan on the path to your call. Don't settle for the perception of others. Be confident in your own feelings. At first glance, my book tour looked to be a failure but proved a success. I didn't complain and I didn't waste my time trying to explain. I simply put one foot in front of the other. After the first week of promotion, when my driver and support staff were cancelled due to higher priority authors, I asked for directions and drove myself to the remaining interviews. I had impromptu opportunities for candid conversations that might otherwise have been stifled by well intended but fast-moving publicity staff. I was able to revisit bookshop staff and learn more about the retail business from their point of view. I spent time with publishing staff and was further educated in the process of getting books into print. A distinguished American author told me later that I learned more on that trip than he had in the publishing of his first five books. It was a wonderful experience.

"The one who dies with the most toys, wins."

– Popular bumper sticker in the 1980's

Shortly after my African book tour, I was a guest speaker at a university event. The professional group sponsoring the occasion had a tradition of honoring birthdays. The master of ceremonies invited those celebrating birthdays that month to speak a few words before we started the day's program. A woman approached the podium and declared that this was going to be the year that she fulfilled her dreams. I sat back and waited anxiously to hear about her calling. Fulfilling one's dream, now that was right up my alley. "This year," she continued, "I will make enough money to buy a brand new car, a bigger house, a better vacation…" the litany went on but I was too stunned to listen. How, I wondered, did she know that these things would make her a better person or provide her life lessons to bring her nearer her own legacy? How did she arrive at these "dreams?" What role did they play in her passion for life?

To be fair, I had just returned from living in Africa, steeped in a culture that treasured the spiritual above the material. Still, the emphasis on physical possessions as an indication of personal success was jolting. My discussions with the group further highlighted cloudy thinking. Removed from their own passions, many were unable to boldly go where their hearts desired. Though well-respected professionals from government, corporate and academic institutions, many seemed disheartened. Their zeal had been hijacked on the road to the right credential, the proper job title, the correct neighborhood, wealth and in many cases, indebtedness. Many had started out with a greater goal but the daily grind took its toll. Several confided that years ago, before marriage, before children and mortgages, they were full of passion and remembered a call. Now, it was impractical. They would not think of making life difficult or uncomfortable for the significant others in their lives.

We need to listen to one another.

– Chaim Potok

By turning our backs on our own call, we deny our loved ones, deceased and living, our gifts, our true legacies. We are intertwined with our families. It is no accident that we are together. Our spouse and children's calls complement and fuel our own. No one call is greater than another's. If we are balanced in our lives, true to our feelings, and living with integrity, no individual call will harm another in the family. Rather, I have noticed quite the opposite. This theory of interconnectedness is not such a stretch for our imaginations. Our ancestors pulled together to build entire communities, created farms and cities, relied on each other and in their efforts developed lasting bonds that are imprinted on our souls today. We are essential cogs in each other's lives. We become each other's advocate but listening is key. Respect must be extended to even the youngest member of the family whose insight can prove valuable or as we found out, even life saving.

Living in Johannesburg was a tenuous proposition as South Africa transitioned from apartheid rule to a new democracy under President Mandela. Apartheid had erected housing along economic and racial lines. These formerly "whites only" neighborhoods were slowly integrating; yet the relative wealth of these areas acted as a magnet to robbers. The fight against apartheid left behind weapons and ammunition now accessible to the growing number of petty thieves. The economy was growing stronger but almost fifty percent of the population lived at or below the poverty level. This volatile situation was intensifying as we approached the end of our work in South Africa.

One Sunday we lounged around the house, enjoying our garden and reading when Joseph, then ten years old, said, "Mom, Dad, I want to go miniature golfing." Ron and I groaned. It had been a busy week and we needed the rest. Miniature golfing was new to Johannesburg. On a Sunday, the recreation center outside the city limits would be packed with young families and screaming kids. We tried to tempt Joseph with movies and books. He was not interested and became more agitated. He said he had a "feeling" we must go away from the neighborhood quickly. That got our attention. We prepared to leave and were soon off in the car.

On our return, a crime scene greeted us. We learned that our forty-year-old neighbor had been killed. Two armed thugs jumped him as he drove into his driveway next door. Shot at point blank range, his body was left on the sidewalk and his vehicle stolen. It was horrible and heart-breaking. His wife and children were devastated; their lovely family shattered. The police said we were lucky to have been away. We mentioned quietly Joseph's premonition of danger, his agitation to get away not only from the house but also from the neighborhood. The police credited our son with sparing our lives as the shooting took place only minutes after we had left. The police believed, without a doubt, that we would have been in danger's way had we been home with our car still in the driveway.

Sharing dreams, visions, observations, premonitions, yearnings, and incidences of synchronicity with our families, we can spontaneously provide a missing puzzle piece to the other. A daughter describes her dream at breakfast. Her mother asks for further clarification and by doing so unintentionally highlights an important and telling detail. A husband's attention to his wife's story of an incident at her office catches a critical synchronicity she had overlooked.

After a television appearance on a health program, the host attended several of my lectures and a number of coaching consultations. Liz had a knack for following her instincts and quickly took to the straightforward ancestor exercises. Soon, she and her husband were exploring a move further east. This had been a dream of theirs for some time and they were emboldened to act. An exploratory trip proved successful and they put their house up for sale. After the sale of the house, Liz felt they should rent a less expensive house until they made their move but worried that downgrading would embarrass the children. She did not want them to feel awkward. I shared the following story.

My husband's and my work, our parents' declining health, and a deep belief in our own callings, have caused us to relocate numerous times. It is never easy to move a family but each transition has its own surprising lessons. Such as when we moved within California from San Diego to the more affluent Orange County and were hit with "sticker shock." Our dollar would not afford us the large house to which we had grown accustomed. Housing would be a cottage, apartment, condominium or townhouse. I empathized with Liz because, in this instance, I too had momentarily felt badly that my son would live in more cramped quarters.

To prepare him for this change, I asked Joseph, of all the many places we had lived, what was his favorite residence? I expected he would site our palatial house on a hillside in Africa or our contemporary view property in Seattle. From there, I thought, we would consider all the strengths and weaknesses of each place and work our way to the smaller yet equally pleasing accommodations we had shared.

Joseph surprised me, as our children often do. Without hesitation he named a tiny studio-like apartment in Washington, D.C. as his favorite. I asked what made it so and he replied, "It was so much fun to be close like that. It was easy to take care of and we spent a lot of time exploring Washington and Virginia and Maryland. It was a big adventure, going from that big house in Africa to this little bird's nest. I really liked it." Needless to say, our move went easily and the new smaller home was perfect.

Given half a chance, our families will astonish us. We are amazingly strong and flexible. We are adventurous in spirit, with pioneers of all varieties in our backgrounds. Find the fun in your family challenges; turn problems into happiness and adventure as you hunt for your unclaimed legacies and ancestral gifts.

All that is gold does not glitter,
Not all those who wander are lost

J.R.R. Tolkien

Home is where the heart is. Home is where I hang my hat. I am home when I am with my family. "Where's home for you?" a stranger asks a fellow traveler on a plane. "Wherever she is," comes the reply, as the man points at his wife."[6] When it boils down to it, we are most at home with those we love, regardless of the location. This is no great surprise given that our early ancestors moved constantly to hunt or shepherd animals, to search for water and wild plants, to provide for their families. Indigenous tribes and European communities relocated en masse to better weather seasonal changes and natural disasters. Our actual survival was once contingent on our mobility. This flexibility of the ancestors is within us still.

Yet, there remains a myth, a yearning to be in one career, one house, for the life of our families within one community or physical location. The reality, however, is that our corporate world requires an adult in the 21st century to change jobs as often as every three years and modify complete careers every ten. Beyond a changing economy and an outdated notion of permanence is a different reality. Home is not a physical building but rather a sense of being on the right course, being in step with the ancestors, living our call, and unraveling our legacies.

On our latest return to the USA, I purchased a cell phone after arriving late to several meetings due to unexpected freeway traffic in our new southern California home. Now I could communicate when delayed

---

[6] From Oxford lecture by Irish poet Seamus Heaney.

or be contacted in an emergency. On reviewing an initial phone bill, I noticed roaming charges for a trip outside my service area. My son Joseph laughed and said, "Just like following a call, Mom. A person may be excited to follow their call but is their dedication strong? Does it come with or without 'roaming charges?' Are they really willing to do what is necessary?"

Joseph makes an important point. He knows first-hand the price of relocations, change and the many adjustments or "roaming charges" that may be required when being true to one's call. Joseph elaborates, "I still don't like to move very much but it is worse, much, much worse to stay put when it is time to go. I can feel it in myself, in school, with friends, when something larger is calling us. Every time we have followed our hearts as a family, I have had awesome experiences. Now in high school, kids tell me how lucky I am to have been raised this way. I always say, I couldn't imagine living any other way!"

CHAPTER TEN

Summary: A Practice of Ancestors

We are not human beings on a spiritual path
But spiritual beings on a human path.

– Jean Shinoda Bolen

Living in spiritual contact with our ancestors is the birthright of every human being. Ancestral contact is a habit that can be developed easily and gently. Over time, this practice of celestial communication becomes a way of life, providing such grace that you will marvel at how you managed to exist before. However, there is one caveat. If you do not do the work, you will not reap the benefits.

What is the work? First, make contact with your ancestors or as the African healers say, "turn your radio on." Honor your lineage through a celebration such as the Ancestor Party. Afterwards dream with intention, then notice what comes through. Be willing to act on the instruction whether it presents itself as remnants of a dream, subtle urgings or a synchronistic event. Demonstrate your willingness, your intent, by acting.

Ancestors want to shape our lives to make them better. Be open and honest with them, remind them of your human limitations and invoke their assistance. Continue to pose your questions and concerns before you sleep. Eventually your relationship with the ancestors will be so natural that you will experience communication throughout your waking moments.

What prevents us from being in relationship with the ancestors? Toxicity in all its forms prevents clear and regular communication. Just like a radio setting filled with static, negative relationships, unhealthy food, and noxious substances clog our own "airwaves" to the divine. Clean up your life in order to tune in or the ancestors may look for better reception elsewhere.

Practice taking the long view by reserving judgment about events being "good" or "bad." Do not analyze guidance coming through. Spiritual guidance and requests may seem odd but avoid jumping to conclusions.

Unless you become again as little children, you cannot enter the kingdom of heaven.

– Matthew 4:4

Lastly, do not take this physical, material world too seriously. Remember the ancestors are playful; have fun with them and enjoy your spiritual guidance. They are only waiting for you to begin. Go with the ancestors and you go with God.

Bibliography

Albom, Mitch, *Tuesdays with Morrie: An Old Man, a Young Man, and Life's Greatest Lesson,* Doubleday Publishing, 1997

Campbell, Susan Schuster, *Called to Heal: African Shamanic Healers,* Lotus Press: Twin Lakes, Wisconsin, 2000

Goodall, Jane, *Reason for Hope,* Warner Books, 1999

Hanh, Thich Nhat, *Going Home: Jesus and Buddha as Brothers,* Riverhead Books, 1999

Houston, Jean, *A Mythic Life : Learning to Live Our Greater Story,* Harper San Francisco, 1997

Kubler-Ross, Elisabeth, *On Death and Dying,* Collier Books, 1970

Rinpoche, Sogyal, *Tibetan Book of Living and Dying,* Harper San Francisco, 1994

Wilbur, Ken, *No Boundary: Eastern and Western Approaches to Personal Growth,* Shambhala Publishing, 1981

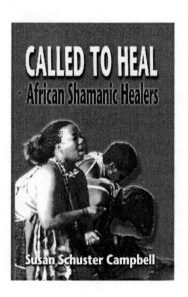